You're Not Alone
UNDERSTANDING AND MANAGING DEPRESSION

Diane Gimpel

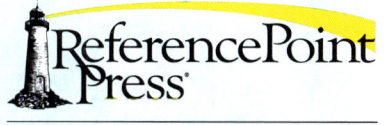

San Diego, CA

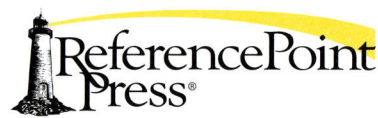

© 2025 ReferencePoint Press, Inc.
Printed in the United States

For more information, contact:
ReferencePoint Press, Inc.
PO Box 27779
San Diego, CA 92198
www.ReferencePointPress.com

ALL RIGHTS RESERVED.
No part of this work covered by the copyright hereon may be reproduced or used in any form or by any means—graphic, electronic, or mechanical, including photocopying, recording, taping, web distribution, or information storage retrieval systems—without the written permission of the publisher.

LIBRARY OF CONGRESS CATALOGING-IN-PUBLICATION DATA

Names: Gimpel, Diane Marczely, author.
Title: You're not alone : understanding and managing depression / by Diane Gimpel.
Description: San Diego, CA : ReferencePoint Press, Inc., 2025. | Includes bibliographical references and index.
Identifiers: LCCN 2023047486 (print) | LCCN 2023047487 (ebook) | ISBN 9781678207762 (library binding) | ISBN 9781678207779 (ebook)
Subjects: LCSH: Depression, Mental--Juvenile literature.
Classification: LCC RC537 .G537 2025 (print) | LCC RC537 (ebook) | DDC 616.85/27--dc23/eng/20231103
LC record available at https://lccn.loc.gov/2023047486
LC ebook record available at https://lccn.loc.gov/2023047487

CONTENTS

Introduction   4
When Depression Strikes Teens

Chapter One   8
What Is Depression?

Chapter Two   16
Who Gets Depression?

Chapter Three   25
Why Are Teens Depressed?

Chapter Four   34
Getting Treatment

Chapter Five   45
Lifestyle Changes Can Help Fight Depression

Source Notes	55
Getting Help and Information	59
Index	61
Picture Credits	64
About the Author	64

INTRODUCTION

When Depression Strikes Teens

M—who uses the pronouns *they/their* and is identified only by an initial for privacy—was in middle school when the trouble started. First, M found it difficult to pay attention in school. Next, M found it difficult to maintain friendships. M was more likely to go to sleep after school than hang out with peers. "I just wanted to be unconscious," M says. "I just sat in my room and cried."[1]

When the COVID-19 pandemic hit in the spring of 2020 and school became a solitary affair experienced through a computer rather than in the school buildings, M stopped paying attention to lessons. That's when M first cut their skin on purpose. "I was mad at myself for not doing homework," M explains. "I was kind of thinking, 'Oh, the pain feels good,' like it was better than being stressed. . . . I wanted to hurt myself with anything."[2]

As seventh grade then became eighth grade and remote learning continued, M, sobbing in bed, told their mom they wanted to die. M got therapy online. Still, self-harm continued. M not only continued to cut but also tried self-strangulation and hitting their head with a barbell, even as they began going to full-day therapy at a mental health clinic. A psychiatrist at the clinic diagnosed M's trouble: depression.

Jamie's Story

As with M, trouble began brewing for Jamie Factor in middle school. She started feeling anxious about socializing with other kids at school. Jamie thought things would change when she got to high school, but they didn't. Jamie was grateful when the pandemic forced learning to happen online in the spring of her freshman year because she was happier at home. However, online school, which continued as she moved into her sophomore year of high school, did not eliminate the need to socialize because sometimes she would have to do group work. "Every day before class I would pray and hope that it would be an easy day—not where there wasn't work but a day when I could work alone,"[3] Jamie writes in a web post.

Even though she preferred being home alone, Jamie signed up to attend a three-week-long summer program out of state after her sophomore year ended. She lasted four days. "I remember arriving and feeling frozen and isolated like I couldn't move,"[4] she notes.

Jamie started therapy and also started taking medication to improve her mood. She started to look forward to going to college—until she didn't. She told her family she was not even going to go to high school anymore. "I was at my breaking point and I wanted to die," Jamie writes. "I talked about jumping off my roof, getting hit by a car, cutting, and so on."[5]

> "I was at my breaking point and I wanted to die."[5]
>
> —Jamie Factor, who was diagnosed with depression in high school

Those thoughts led Jamie to get more intensive therapy, new medications, and a new therapist. Like M, Jamie was diagnosed with depression. Jamie also was diagnosed with anxiety.

Madison Jo's Story

Madison Jo Sieminski was a sophomore in high school when she began feeling unhealthy—older than M and Jamie were when their mental health began changing. "I noticed I was never fully myself," Madison Jo writes on a blog. "There has been someone inside of my head telling me to constantly worry and hold back from everything. Did I listen? Of course I did. I withdrew and shrank into myself."[6]

In her post, Madison Jo talks about sleeping all the time—staying in bed late into the afternoon, and, even after waking, being unable to stay awake for longer than thirty minutes at a time. "Most days I have little motivation to do anything and it is mentally and physically draining," she explains. "Lying in bed wanting to get up but not being able to is a horrible feeling."[7]

Like M and Jamie, Madison Jo sought professional help and was diagnosed as having depression. And like Jamie, she also was diagnosed with anxiety.

Depression Is a Medical Problem

Depression is a mental illness. In other illnesses, the heart, lungs, skin, or bones might not be working properly. In a mental illness, the organ that is not working properly is the brain. Like what other illnesses do, a mental illness affects a person's everyday life. How-

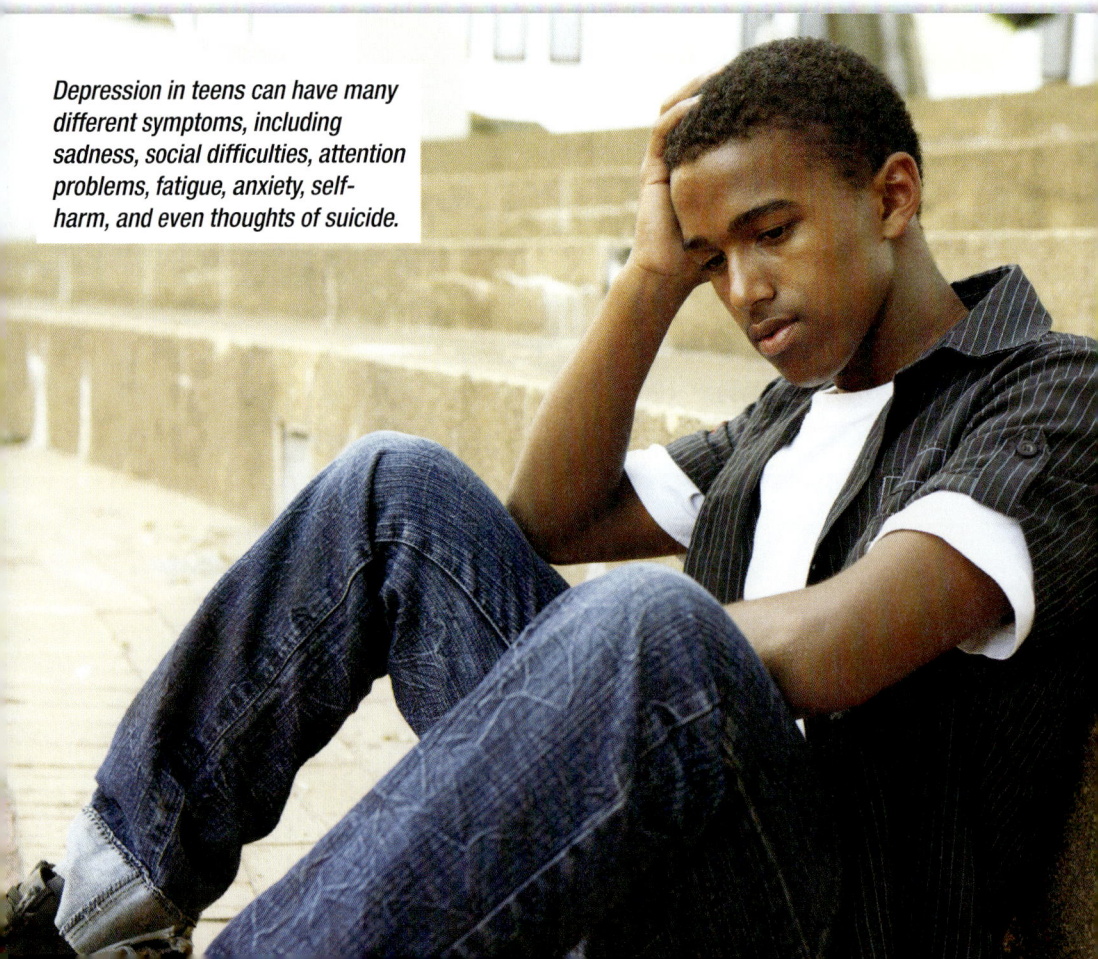

Depression in teens can have many different symptoms, including sadness, social difficulties, attention problems, fatigue, anxiety, self-harm, and even thoughts of suicide.

ever, unlike other illnesses, someone who has a mental illness might not realize it right away because the person might not feel physical pain, although some people with depression do.

> "Most days I have little motivation to do anything and it is mentally and physically draining. Lying in bed wanting to get up but not being able to is a horrible feeling."[7]
>
> —Madison Jo Sieminski, a teen diagnosed with depression

Someone with depression might not have fun anymore doing things that used to be fun. A person with depression might feel tired a lot—like Madison Jo—or might struggle to make decisions that used to be easy to make. On the other hand, a person with depression may make decisions too quickly on matters that require more thought or may start making unhealthy choices.

In other words, depression can affect different people in different ways. A mental health professional must evaluate their behavior and thoughts before diagnosing whether they have depression. Once that happens, treatment can begin.

CHAPTER ONE

What Is Depression?

Depression, according to the American Psychiatric Association (APA), is a mood disorder that is serious, common, and treatable. The illness affects the way someone feels, thinks, and behaves. Because of that, a person with depression can have trouble functioning from one day to the next.

Having depression—the mood disorder—is not the same thing as being sad. Someone who is sad because of the death of a friend or loved one, for example, might find the sadness coming and going as good memories ease the feelings of loss from time to time. Someone who has depression, on the other hand, will feel sadness steadily and almost exclusively for a long period of time—two weeks or more. In addition, those who are sad about a loss don't feel bad about themselves, but those with depression often feel worthless, which can lead them to think about ending their lives to end their painful thoughts. However, sometimes an event that causes sadness can lead to depression.

Someone who has depression, according to the APA, experiences certain symptoms for two weeks or more, and these symptoms negatively affect the person's ability to function. Among the symptoms are sadness, loss of interest in activities that used to bring enjoyment, eating more—or less—than usual, sleeping more—or less—than usual, trouble focusing or making decisions, and suicidal thinking.

Teens and Depression

Teens with depression may demonstrate one or more of a variety of symptoms. They may spend more time alone, and they may spend more time on their computers or handheld electronics instead of spending time with friends. The difficulties they experience with just getting through each day may mean they start performing poorly at school or in sports or other activities. They might cry more easily or act out angrily. They might be extra irritable. They may use drugs or alcohol to try to feel different, or they may stop caring about the way they look.

Some of the symptoms of depression in teens also include behaviors that adults expect from teens, such as acting moody and irritable. Also, teens sometimes have trouble processing their thoughts or expressing them to adults. Nonetheless, a teen who is moodier, more irritable and isolated, and sadder than usual or for a longer time than usual might be depressed.

Desperately Sad

A number of different types of depression exist. Major depression—also known as major depressive disorder—is "one of the most common psychiatric disorders of childhood and adolescence,"[8] according to Sandra Mullen, who specializes in child and adolescent psychiatry at the Virginia Treatment Center for Children. Major depression usually involves sadness, irritability, lack of interest in activities that previously brought pleasure, isolation, and self-loathing. Those symptoms must interfere with everyday life and must persist for more than two weeks for a diagnosis of major depression. A teen can be diagnosed with a mild, moderate, or severe case of this illness, depending on the severity of the symptoms.

Another common form of depression in young people is persistent depressive disorder. Boston Children's Hospital notes that 11 percent of Americans between the ages of thirteen and eighteen have major depressive disorder or persistent depressive disorder. With this disorder, the symptoms continue for a long time—a year or more. One fifteen-year-old patient who was being treated

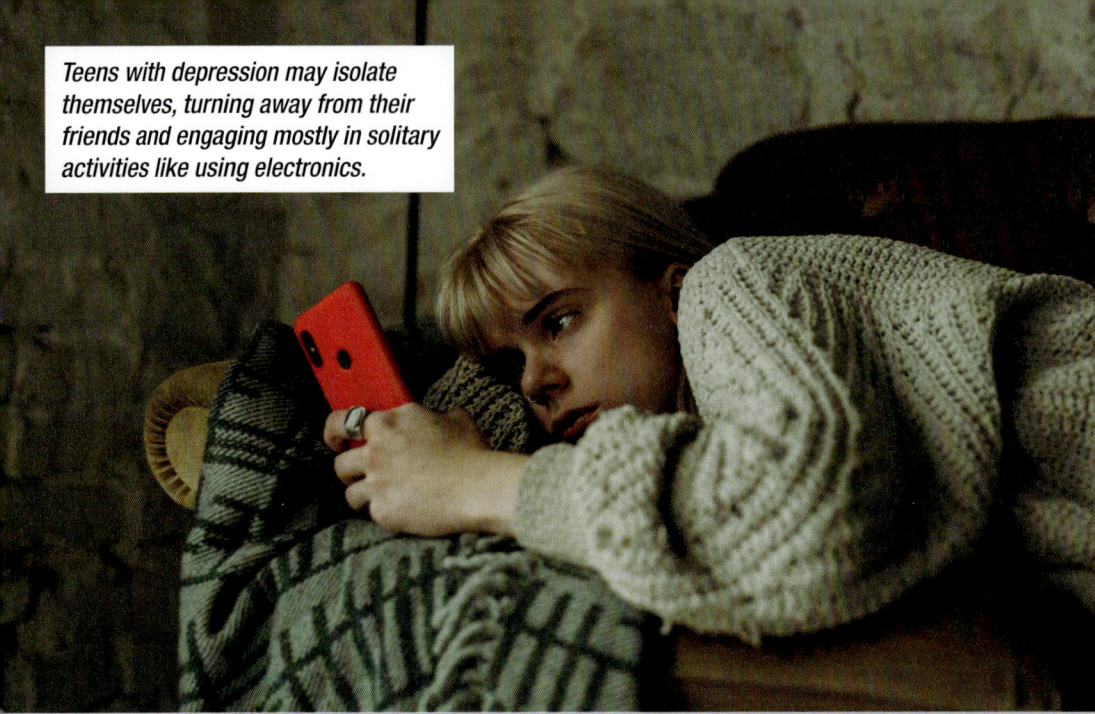

Teens with depression may isolate themselves, turning away from their friends and engaging mostly in solitary activities like using electronics.

for major depressive disorder felt sad, couldn't feel pleasure, and had trouble falling asleep, according to an article Mullen wrote for the journal *Mental Health Clinician*. The teen's grades were going down. In addition, Mullen wrote, "the patient has not been able to reestablish relationships with friends and feels there is no longer any point in living or attending college. . . . Self-injurious behavior, including cutting bilateral forearms and hips 'as a way to not feel numb,' is a daily occurrence."[9]

Change of Seasons

Some teens get seasonal affective disorder (SAD). With SAD, the symptoms of depression show up as the days get shorter in the fall and start to go away when the days get longer in the spring. The disorder typically shows up in the late teen years, according to the National Institutes of Health, and it shows up much more often in girls than in boys. When teens experience SAD, their symptoms can differ from those of adults with the disorder. For example, teens might be irritable or angry instead of sad and depressed, or they may sleep a lot instead of suffering from insomnia, as many adults with the disorder do.

More than a million people nineteen years old and younger have SAD, according to Children's National Hospital in Washington, DC. Among them is Meg McCarney. She became irritable and wanted to sleep a lot when SAD would afflict her in the middle of each September, beginning in high school. "Normally I'm an involved and engaged person but, in the fall, my passion for activities that I love becomes something that I have to struggle every day to hold on to," she explains. "I have difficulty regulating my movements and keeping my life in order. There's a noticeable shift in the way I behave as soon as depression arrives for the season. I get frustrated and upset for seemingly no reason. Dragging myself out of bed in the morning becomes grueling."[10]

> "Normally I'm an involved and engaged person but, in the fall, my passion for activities that I love becomes something that I have to struggle every day to hold on to."[10]
>
> —Meg McCarney, who was diagnosed with SAD as a teen

Irritable and Angry

Unlike SAD, which primarily occurs in adults, disruptive mood dysregulation disorder (DMDD) is a type of depression that mainly affects children and teens. Young people with this condition are irritable and angry for a long time. They throw a lot of really bad temper tantrums, during which they may hurt other people and damage things. Because of these symptoms and behaviors, those who have DMDD often are in trouble at home and at school.

Owen, now in his teens, was diagnosed with DMDD when he was eight. The diagnosis came about five years after trouble started. Owen would throw tantrums that were more extreme than most toddler tantrums. The tantrums didn't stop as he grew older, and they got in the way of Owen's family life, school life, and social life. "I had a lot of anger and anxiety," he says. "It was hard to control. Feelings of being friendless and depressed didn't help either."[11]

Physical and Mental Distress

Premenstrual dysphoric disorder (PMDD) is a depressive disorder that affects around 5 percent of girls who have gone through puberty

Is There a Blood Test for Depression?

Doctors often prescribe a blood test when a patient has symptoms of depression to rule out causes for those symptoms other than depression, such as low blood sugar or anemia. No blood test exists that detects depression—at least, not yet—but scientists are trying to develop one.

Scientists found that many people with depression had low levels of a blood protein called mature brain-derived neurotrophic factor, according to a 2021 story published by PsychCentral. Another finding, described in the same story, is that many people with major depressive disorder had low levels of an enzyme called ethanolamine phosphate in their blood. Neither of these findings have led to a definitive blood test for depression, although research continues.

To date, the best way to determine whether someone has depression is to go to a doctor who can evaluate the person's symptoms. Usually, that person will undergo a physical exam and lab tests to rule out explanations for those symptoms other than depression.

---

and some women as well. The disorder causes physical discomfort, including bloating and headaches, before a girl gets her period each month. It also causes emotional problems such as depression and irritability. As is the case with other types of depression, the symptoms of PMDD interfere with the everyday life of those who have it. The fact that the symptoms are so severe that they disrupt daily functioning is what makes PMDD different from premenstrual syndrome (PMS), a more common condition that affects women a week or two before their periods and causes physical symptoms like bloating and emotional symptoms like irritability.

Casey Clark was in high school when she realized her premenstrual symptoms were so extreme that she couldn't function normally. Besides excruciating cramps, Casey could not concentrate in class and was irritable. Sometimes, she says, she even felt like she wanted to die.

People like Casey and others who have depression may realize something is wrong with the way they think or behave, but they will not know what it is or what to do about it without help. To find a way to cope with the problem, a person must first get a diagnosis of what the problem is. That involves visiting a doctor or a mental health professional. The visit can be—but does not have to be—to a psychiatrist, who is a medical doctor who specializes in diagnosing and treating mental illness. A family doctor or a pediatrician can diagnose depression, too, as can psychologists, mental health counselors, clinical social workers, and psychiatric nurses.

Diagnosing Depression

During an appointment to determine whether a teen has depression, the health care provider will do a physical exam to look for a physical explanation for the depression symptoms. The health care provider also will ask a lot of questions and may have the teen complete a questionnaire. Some questions will be about the teen's feelings. For example, the questions might ask how often and how long the teen feels those emotions, and how those feelings affect the teen's daily functioning, such as getting up in the morning, socializing, keeping clean, doing schoolwork, eating, and sleeping. Other questions will have to do with medications the teen takes, past medical history, and family medical history. The doctor will ask these things because some medications cause symptoms like those of depression, and some health problems can cause depression-like symptoms. Family medical history is important because sometimes depression can run in families.

In addition, the doctor may order a blood test. A blood test can show whether the teen has nutritional deficiencies that are linked with depression, such as levels of B vitamins or vitamin D that are too low.

A blood test also can show whether the teen has a problem other than depression that is causing depression symptoms. Caffeine withdrawal and dehydration can cause depression-like symptoms, as can low blood sugar, mononucleosis, some thyroid problems, anemia, and even some cancers. If the blood test does not show the existence of a condition that could cause depression symptoms, then that could be evidence that the teen has depression.

Why It's Difficult to Diagnose Depression in Teens

The bottom line is, no one medical test exists—like a blood test or a urine test, for example—that can say for sure that someone has depression. That is one reason depression is difficult to diagnose in anyone, let alone teens.

> "As my thoughts became darker, scarier, and more erratic, I became quieter and more aloof."[12]
>
> —Kimberly Zapata, who had depression as a teen

Even with the available diagnosing methodologies, such as questionnaires and interviews conducted by health professionals, depression can be difficult to diagnose in teens. Some of the difficulty has to do with teens keeping their feelings to themselves. Kimberly Zapata says she felt "a deep, permeating sadness" that left her exhausted, in physical pain, and hopeless. "I never spoke to anyone, though. As my thoughts became darker, scarier, and more erratic, I became quieter and more aloof,"[12] she recalls.

Teens stay quiet for various reasons. They might not understand what is going on. Teens also may stay quiet or minimize their symptoms because they are afraid whatever they admit to a doctor or therapist will be repeated to their parents or guardians. Some also

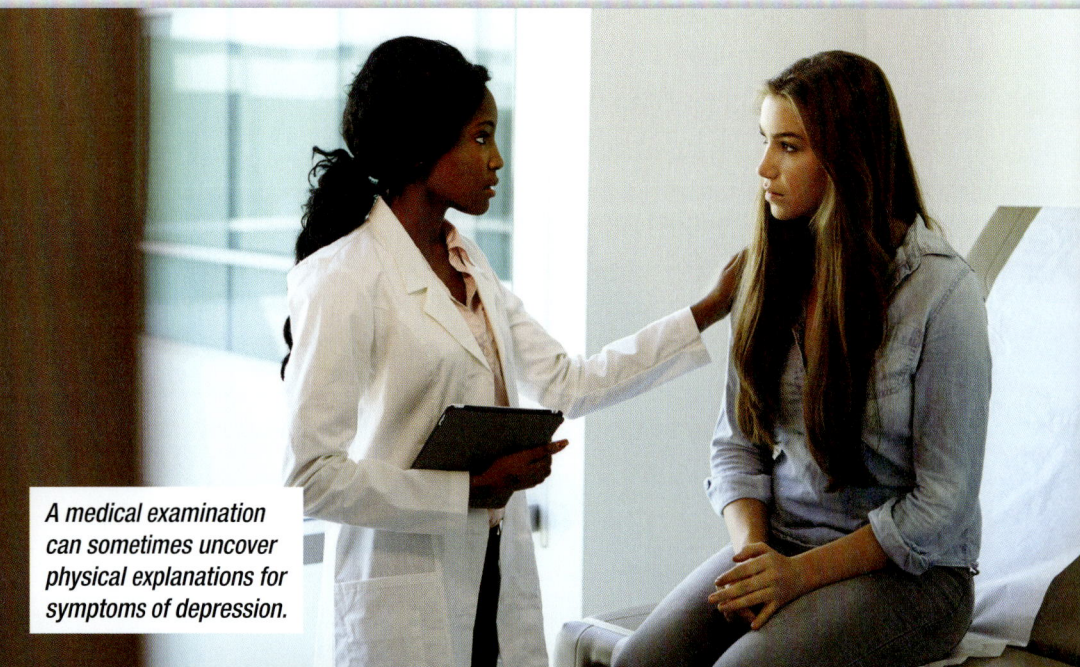

A medical examination can sometimes uncover physical explanations for symptoms of depression.

What's Normal for Teens—and What Isn't

Adolescents who are developing normally can sleep late, get irritated easily, and be moody. Adolescents with depression can behave similarly. What's the difference?

In a 2022 article, Alissa Briggs, a psychologist who works for the University of Kentucky's adolescent medicine program, pointed out some differences between normal adolescent behavior and the behavior of a depressed adolescent. Briggs wrote that it is normal for a teen to overreact to things occasionally, but it's not normal for a teen to be moody or irritable all the time. It's not uncommon for teens to resist hanging out with their families, but there is cause for concern when teens stop hanging out with their friends. Teens often are tired in the morning and want to sleep late on weekends, but a teen who refuses to get out of bed in the morning or sleeps all the time may be depressed. A teen giving up playing baseball to join the cast of the spring musical probably isn't a sign of depression, but a teen who used to be happily involved in activities and no longer does much of anything could be depressed.

fear that the health care professional will discount their feelings. Also, teens don't want to think of themselves as ill or crazy. They don't want to be different from their peers or considered weak.

Another problem with diagnosis is that those around the depressed adolescent might mistake that person's behavior for normal teen behavior. Parents may see their child's mood, socializing, sleeping, or eating change and think the shift is part of a typical phase their child will outgrow. Sometimes they are right, but sometimes they are not.

Further complicating the matter is that depression is different in different people. "There are more than 1,500 possible combinations of symptoms that meet criteria for a depressive disorder, meaning that patients can share the same diagnosis and have no symptoms in common. As a result, depression often gets overlooked and undertreated,"[13] according to New York University.

Nonetheless, plenty of teens, with the help of their parents or guardians, recognize problem signs and seek diagnosis. Because of that, it has become clear that many American teens have depression, and the incidence of it is on the rise.

CHAPTER TWO

Who Gets Depression?

Anyone can have depression, including teens. The National Institute of Mental Health estimates that more than 20 percent of American adolescents have experienced depression during their teen years. That is one out of every five teens. Worldwide, 1.1 percent of people between the ages of ten and fourteen and 2.8 percent of people between the ages of fifteen and nineteen suffer from depression, according to the World Health Organization.

Depression Among Teens Is on the Rise

Not only do a lot of teens experience depression, but also the incidence of depression in that age group is going up in the United States. It is a cause for alarm, according to US surgeon general Vivek H. Murthy. In a 2021 advisory, Murthy wrote, "Recent national surveys of young people have shown alarming increases in the prevalence of certain mental health challenges—in 2019, one in three high school students and half of female students reported persistent feelings of sadness or hopelessness, an overall increase of 40% from 2009."[14]

A March 2022 article in the *Journal of Adolescent Health* called attention to this increase. In 2009, 8.1 percent of the almost 168,000 American teens who participated in the National Survey of Drug Use and Health reported being depressed, write Sylia Wilson and Nathalie M. Dumornay of the University of Minnesota's Institute of Child Development. In 2019, that rate increased to 15.8 percent. "These findings are consistent with other recent . . . studies in the United States and the world in highlighting a potential adolescent mental health crisis,"[15] Wilson and Dumornay note.

Wilson and Dumornay are among many people in science, health care, and government who have examined the problem. In 2021, a survey conducted by the US Centers for Disease Control and Prevention (CDC) found that 44 percent of high school student respondents reported "persistent feelings of sadness or hopelessness."[16] In 2009, 26 percent of respondents to the CDC survey had reported such feelings.

Fame Does Not Make You Immune to Depression

Depression is an illness that anyone can get, no matter how old they are, where they live, or how famous they are. In fact, several celebrities have revealed that they had depression when they were teens. Among them are US Olympic gymnast and medalist Simone Biles; recording artists Billie Eilish, Justin Bieber, and Lady Gaga; and actor Sophie Turner.

Although some may think that fame and riches would make a person immune to depression, that was not the case for Bieber. Bieber, who was 15 when he had his first hit song, has been public with his mental health challenges, for which he sought help from professionals. Bieber spoke to his fans directly about the issue in a September 2019 Instagram post in which he wrote, "It's hard to get out of bed in the morning when you are overwhelmed with your life, your past, job, responsibilities, emotions, your family, finances, your relationships. When it feels like there's trouble after trouble after trouble. . . . Sometimes it can get to the point where you don't even want to live anymore."[17] In the 2020 YouTube documentary *Justin Bieber: The Next Chapter,* Bieber talks about how he was feeling as a teen, trying to navigate life in the spotlight. "Man, I think that there were times when I was really, really suicidal," Bieber recalls.

The Struggles of LGBTQ Young People

In January 2022 thirteen-year-old AJ Frederick tried to kill himself after months of battling thoughts of suicide. AJ is gay and transgender. Even though he was in therapy, the pressures of school and living in a state controlled by lawmakers who are unfriendly to people like him deepened his depression.

AJ told his parents about his suicide attempt. They immediately got more treatment for him than his therapy appointments could provide. "I realized that I don't want to die, and I realized that I need help," he says.

AJ is just one among many LGBTQ young people whose depression has taken a potentially deadly turn. LGBTQ young people think about suicide more than their non-LGBTQ peers. According to the CDC, almost 50 percent of LGBTQ high school students considered suicide and more than 25 percent attempted it in 2021. The numbers are far lower in the heterosexual population: 14 percent of heterosexual students considered suicide and 5 percent attempted it, the CDC says. Experts say that discrimination and family rejection are among the factors that lead to the difference.

Quoted in Orion Rummler,. "LGBTQ People on Hope After Thoughts of Suicide," *Teen Vogue*, May 12, 2022. www.teenvogue.com.

"Like, really, like, man, is this pain ever gonna go away? It was so consistent. The pain was so consistent. I was just suffering, right? So, I'm just like, man, I would rather not feel this than feel this."[18]

Feeling Miserable and Unworthy

Like Bieber, Eilish rose to fame quickly as a teen but succumbed to depression even though she had accomplished what many work for decades to achieve—but never do. "I was 14, 15 and then 16 touring for the first time and I was also very depressed because I was 14, 15, 16, as you are," she said on a 2021 *Smartless* podcast hosted by Jason Bateman, Sean Hayes, and Will Arnett. She explained,

> You're just doing so much and I also was new to fame and suddenly I didn't have any friends because I was famous and I was leaving all the time and it was weird. It was really weird. . . . I really hated everything about it and I felt stupid

because I was like, wow, I have this thing that is really cool and people would kill for this and I don't like it at all. I was also forgetting that I was really, really depressed and that could make you hate almost anything.[19]

Although the fame that came with her success added to her depression, Eilish says the catalyst for the depression was being forced to stop working with a competitive dance company after she ruptured a growth plate in her hip when she was thirteen. "I think that's when the depression started," she told *Rolling Stone* magazine. "I went through a whole self-harming phase—we don't have to go into it. But the gist of it was, I felt like I deserved to be in pain. It's funny. When anyone else thinks about Billie Eilish at 14, they think of all the good things that happened. But all I can think of is how miserable I was. How completely distraught and confused. Thirteen to 16 was pretty rough."[20]

Like Bieber and Eilish, actor Turner was young—fourteen—when she began filming the cable television role for which she

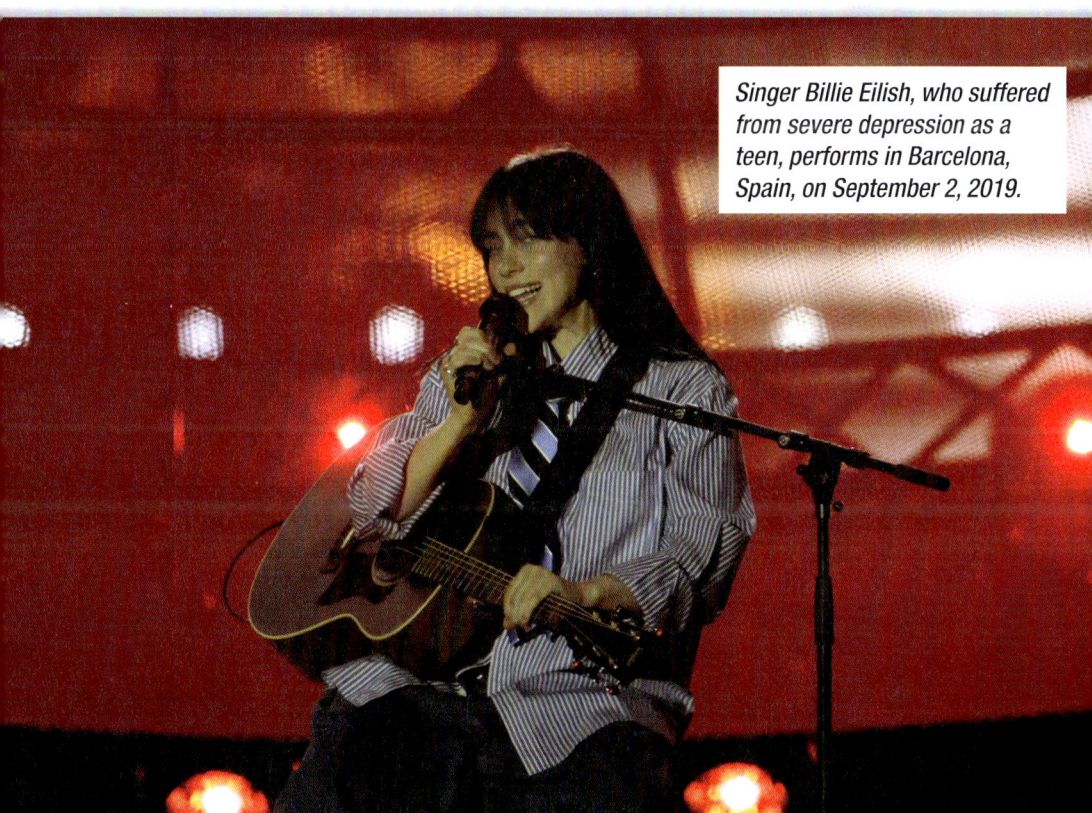

Singer Billie Eilish, who suffered from severe depression as a teen, performs in Barcelona, Spain, on September 2, 2019.

More Girls Are Depressed than Boys: Why?

Five percent or less of both boys and girls are likely to be diagnosed with depression or another mood disorder. When those children become teens, however, the girls have a 14 to 20 percent chance of being diagnosed with a mood disorder, a percentage that is more than double that for boys. Experts attribute that difference, in part, to girls maturing emotionally and physically faster than boys in an environment that has a lot of triggering stressors, like social media.

During puberty, the production of estrogen in girls increases. Estrogen increases the immune system's response to bodily stressors, which can be good at keeping a girl healthy. However, when girls experience a lot of stressors—such as emotional reactions to likes or dislikes on social media—their immune system can overreact and behave as if the body is being harmed physically. "When girls experience overwhelming social and emotional stressors at the same time that estrogen is coming onboard during puberty, this can exacerbate the ill effects of stress on health and development," says Donna Jackson Nakazawa, author of *Girls on the Brink: Helping Our Daughters Thrive in an Era of Increased Anxiety, Depression, and Social Media.*

Quoted in Elissa Strauss, "Why Today's Girls Are So Anxious and Depressed," *CNN*, October 11, 2022. www.cnn.com.

---

gained fame: Sansa Stark in HBO's *Game of Thrones*. Negative social media commentary led her to negative thinking and, eventually, suicidal thinking. "I don't think I viewed myself as worthy of anything that I was doing,"[21] she says. During that period of her life, Turner would "cry and cry and cry over just getting changed and having to put on clothes and be like, 'I can't do this. I can't go outside. I have nothing that I want to do,'"[22] she remembers.

> "I don't think I viewed myself as worthy of anything that I was doing."[21]
>
> —Sophie Turner, actor

Different Types of Struggles

In Biles's case, a traumatic episode triggered depression. Biles was a teen when she became one of the hundreds of American gymnasts who were assaulted by Larry Nassar, the doctor for the US women's Olympic gymnastics team.

When news of Nassar's crimes became public, Biles at first denied the doctor had assaulted her. Eventually, she revealed the abuse to her mother and her agent, and then succumbed to depression. In the 2021 Facebook Watch documentary series *Simone vs. Herself*, Biles talks about how she felt during this time:

> I was, like, super depressed, I didn't want to leave my room, and I didn't want to go anywhere, and I kind of, like, just shut everybody out. . . . I remember being on the phone with my agent and stuff and I remember telling my mom and my agent that I slept all the time and it's because sleeping was, like, basically better than offing myself. It was, like, my way to escape reality and sleeping was, like, the closest to death to me at that point, so I just slept all the time.[23]

For Lady Gaga, whose birth name is Stefani Germanotta, depression set in during middle school. In an interview about raising her famous daughter, Cynthia Germanotta blames bullying. "In

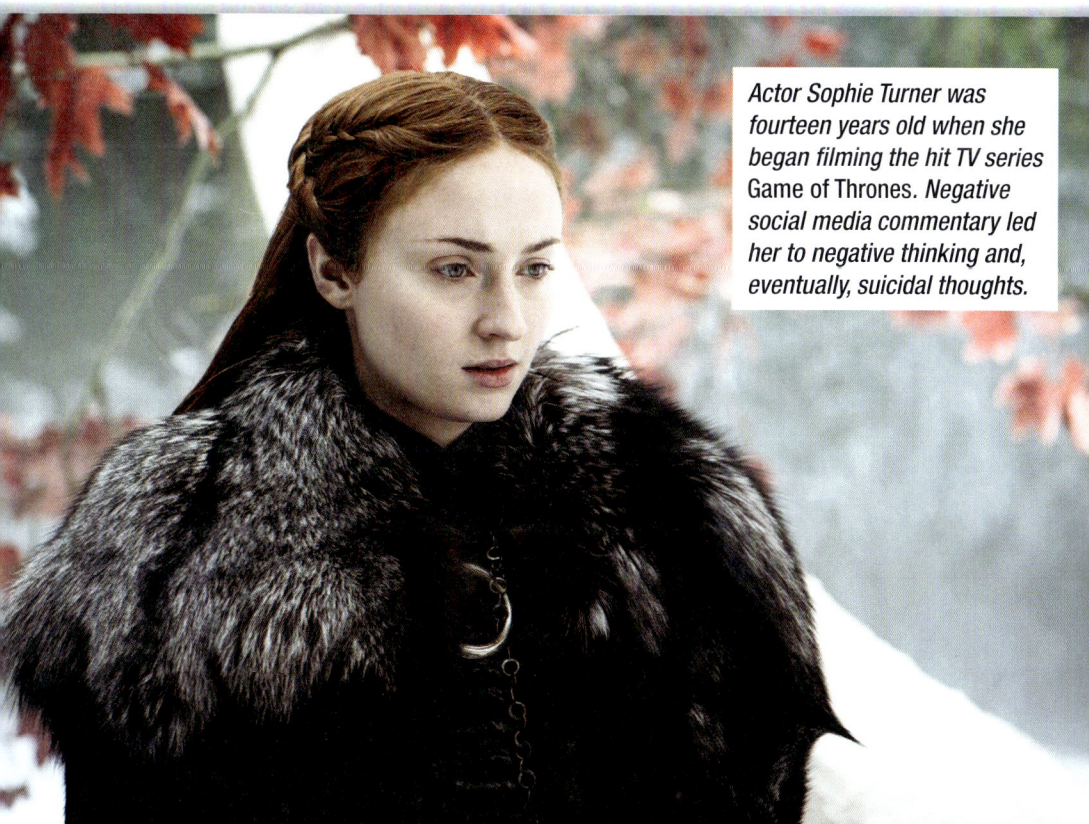

Actor Sophie Turner was fourteen years old when she began filming the hit TV series Game of Thrones. *Negative social media commentary led her to negative thinking and, eventually, suicidal thoughts.*

middle school, because she was unique, she started experiencing a lot of struggles," Germanotta says. "You know, feeling isolated from events. Humiliated. Taunted. And she would start to question herself and become doubtful of her own abilities. And that's when she developed depression."[24] Now in her thirties, the mental health condition continues to be a factor in Lady Gaga's life, and she does not always experience happiness like those without depression do. "I have clinical depression. There's something going on in my brain where the dopamine and serotonin are not firing the same way, and I can't get there. . . . I'm not standing over here with a flag going, 'I'm all healed, everything's perfect.' It's not; it's a fight all the time. I still work on myself constantly. I have bad days, I have good days."[25]

> "It's a fight all the time. I still work on myself constantly. I have bad days, I have good days."[25]
>
> —Lady Gaga, recording artist

Risk Factors for Teen Depression

Although teens can have depression regardless of their wealth, fame, or gender, some factors make a teen more likely to have the illness. One factor is being female. Teen girls are three times more likely than teen boys to have been depressed in the recent past, according to a 2019 study by the Pew Research Center. Twenty percent of teenage girls had a depressive episode during the survey year compared to 7 percent of teenage boys. Pew's findings are backed up by a 2021 study by experts in adolescent depression from around the world. This study noted that being female is one of the risk factors for depression.

That international study also identified other factors that contribute to teen depression. These factors include family history of depression, exposure to bullying, a negative family environment, and physical illness or disability. Other factors are loss of a loved one, exposure to trauma, substance abuse, social difficulties, academic stress, poverty, and low self-esteem.

One person who experienced a couple of those risk factors was Sam. Sam was a high school athlete who was injured during her sophomore year, which meant she couldn't play sports. The risk factors Sam met were being female and suffering a physical disability. "Being an athlete offered Sam a strong sense of self; without that in her life, the feelings of isolation were only magnified. She began spiraling into depression and had recurring thoughts about hurting herself,"[26] according to a story in *Boston* magazine.

Other Risk Factors

Teens with some other characteristics may be at risk too. Having another mental health condition, such as anxiety or attention-deficit/hyperactivity disorder, puts a teen at risk of having depression. Teens who drink too much alcohol, which is a depressant, or abuse other drugs or nicotine, also risk getting depression. Other risk factors include having a learning disability, being overly dependent on others, and being pessimistic.

One of the biggest risk factors for teen depression, experts note, is being LGBTQ. Fifty-eight percent of the more than thirty-four thousand LGBTQ youth who responded to a 2022 poll by the

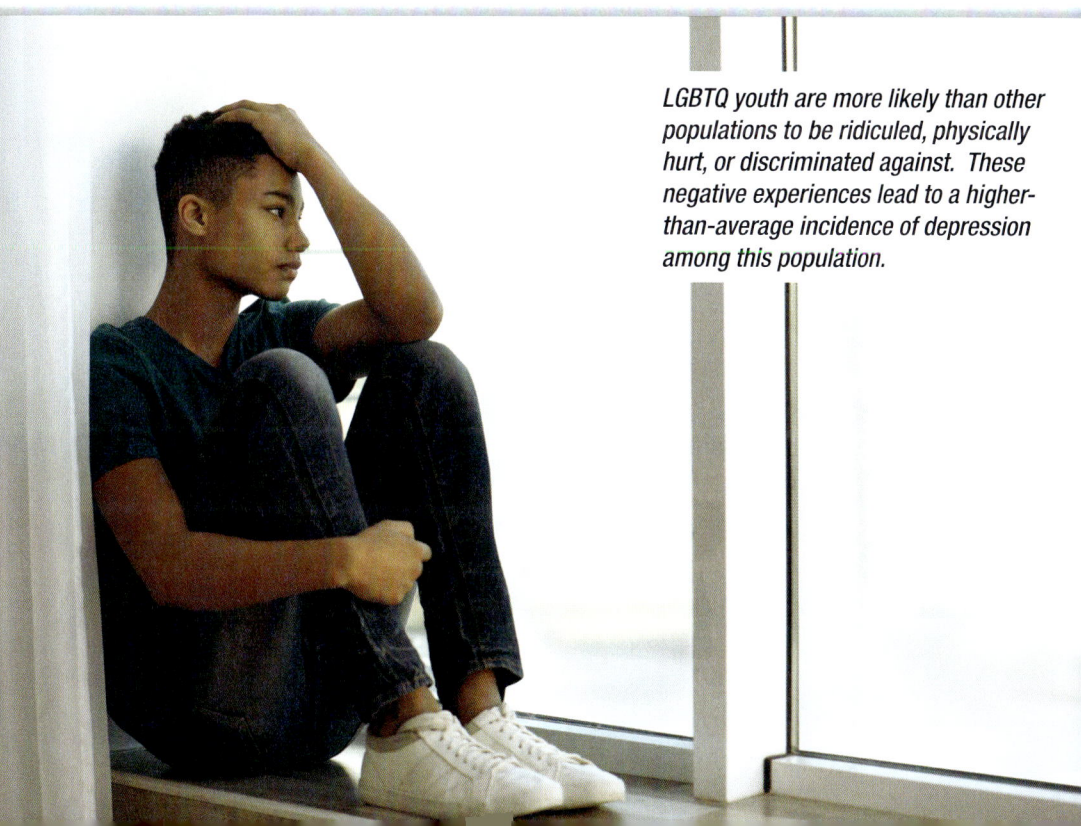

LGBTQ youth are more likely than other populations to be ridiculed, physically hurt, or discriminated against. These negative experiences lead to a higher-than-average incidence of depression among this population.

Trevor Project, which is a suicide prevention and mental health organization for LGBTQ young people, said they had depressive symptoms. Forty-five percent of those polled said they had suicidal ideations (thoughts). According to the CDC, 69 percent of LGBTQ youth reported feeling persistently sad and hopeless—a symptom of depression—during 2021.

Being LGBTQ does not cause depression, but being subjected to negative treatment by peers or others can bring on depression. LGBTQ individuals are sometimes ridiculed or physically or sexually hurt, or they may be denied jobs or services offered to other people. Rejection by family also heightens the risk for depression.

Risk Factors Versus Causes

Just because someone has a risk factor for depression doesn't mean the person will become depressed. Not all girls are depressed, for example. Scientists only know that more girls have depression than boys. Conversely, someone can be wealthy, male, physically able, and academically gifted; have lots of friends and a great family; and have no issues with substance abuse, trauma, bullying, or loss of loved ones—and still have depression.

Science indicates it is likely a combination of internal risk factors (such as genetics or physical illness) and external risk factors (such as bullying, social isolation, or substance abuse) that causes depression. Some scientists say recent developments like social media and the COVID-19 pandemic, which would fit in the category of external risk factors, are also causes of depression.

CHAPTER THREE

Why Are Teens Depressed?

There are many possible causes of teen depression. Some relatively recent developments—the COVID-19 pandemic, social media use, and the falling age of puberty—may be behind the increase in the number of young people experiencing mental illness. In general, though, the interaction between social factors, emotional factors, and biological and chemical factors lies at the heart of mental illness.

Brain Chemistry

Scientists used to think that people became depressed because they had low levels of neurotransmitters—chemicals that carry messages from one nerve cell in the brain to another. If that were true, then people with depression would feel better immediately when they took certain prescription medications that increase those chemicals. However, that's not what happens, according to Harvard Medical School. A depressed person has to take the medication daily for a few weeks before mood improves. Scientists think the reason it takes a few weeks for people to feel better is because the medications help the brain create new nerve cells and nerve cell connections as well as improve message delivery. In other words, depression involves both chemistry and biology.

This can also be seen in the way hormonal changes happen in the brain. During puberty, as the human body changes from a child's to an adolescent's, hormonal changes can affect the production of the brain chemicals that influence mood. Drops in estrogen, which is the female hormone, or testosterone, which is the male hormone, can lead to depression.

Studies also show that the early onset of puberty can lead to depression, especially in girls. The average age for puberty is eleven for girls and twelve for boys, but that age has been decreasing since the late twentieth century. Recently, scientists have said it is not uncommon for puberty to start around eight in girls and around nine in boys. That decrease in age does not seem to have a singular cause, although some point to obesity, stress, and the environment.

Genetics

Although brain chemicals such as the hormones released during puberty can have an impact on depression, so can a person's DNA—that is, the traits inherited from parents, grandparents, and other blood relatives. Depression can—but does not always—run in families. In a blog post, Madison Jo Sieminski, who was diagnosed with depression and anxiety in high school, says her mother had depression. "Growing up, seeing my mom upset or having a bad day always broke my heart. It took her years to better herself and she still has hard days,"[27] she explains.

> "Both of my parents and several of their siblings have had depression. Knowing that genetics is commonly considered one of many underlying causes for depression, they suspected that my brother and I would get what we now call 'The Family Depression' as well."[28]
>
> —Jack Bliss, who was diagnosed with depression in high school

In the family of Jack Bliss, who was diagnosed with depression in high school, it was not just one relative who had depression—it was several. "Both of my parents and several of their siblings have had depression. Knowing that genetics is commonly considered one of many underlying causes for depression, they suspected that my brother and I would get what we now call 'The Family Depression' as well. They were not wrong,"[28] Bliss says.

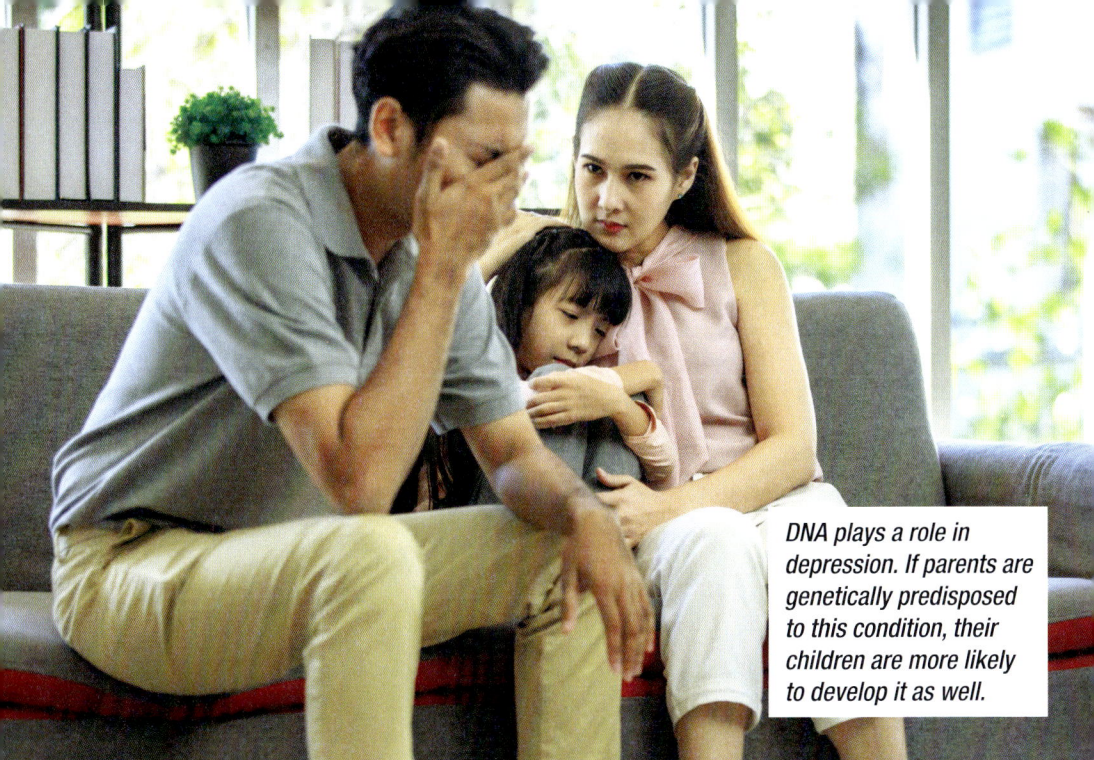

DNA plays a role in depression. If parents are genetically predisposed to this condition, their children are more likely to develop it as well.

Actress Kristen Bell also attributed her depression, which manifested in her teen years, to genetic factors related to serotonin, a chemical that affects a person's mood. "My mom sat me down when I was probably 18 and said, 'There is a serotonin imbalance in our family line and it can often be passed from female to female,'" Bell says. "My mom's a nurse and she had the wherewithal to recognize it in herself."[29]

The fact that depression can run in families suggests that something genetic is afoot in causing the disorder. Researchers have found that people with depression who also have a family history of the disorder have a different genetic structure than those who have depression and do not have a family history of it. Additionally, scientists have found that young people are more likely to develop the disorder if multiple generations of their family have had it. However, no single gene or genetic marker has been found that causes depression, which means a genetic test cannot be created yet for the illness.

Researchers suggest that several genes or genetic variations could combine to cause depression. Some genes that could be

Struggling to Cope During the COVID-19 Pandemic

In addition to causing physical illness in millions of people, COVID-19 triggered depression and anxiety in people who struggled to cope with the isolation required when schools, businesses, and government offices were shut down to try to stop the spread of the disease. Among those who faced mental health struggles were teens.

One young person who talked about the struggle was Christopher Cummings of Michigan, who was in twelfth grade during the first year of the pandemic. "I'd say I've learned not to really take human interaction for granted because honestly, I think the isolation is starting to take a toll on me," Cummings admitted.

Another twelfth grader who struggled with the isolation was Matthew Lyons of Massachusetts. "As much as I love being home, working on my computer, watching movies, nothing can replace the feeling you get when you're out with friends, when you're with family, when you're taking a walk in the park, when you're doing something that's outside and with someone else," Lyons explained.

The bottom line: the pandemic was stressful on young people. "An adult goes through a lot of stress, but being in a pandemic at the age of 13 actually can take a toll," said Davina Doshi, who was an eighth grader in Michigan during the pandemic.

Quoted in Rawan Elbaba and Leila Jackson, "How Teens Adapted and Changed During the Pandemic," *PBS NewsHour*, March 25, 2021. www.pbs.org.

---

involved in depression are the ones that control neurotransmitters—the chemicals that carry brain signals from one nerve cell to another. Some might impact brain nerve cell growth.

Stress That Results from Trauma

The genetic predisposition a person may have for depression is not a guarantee the person will get it. It may be like a switch that exists but is on the "off" setting. Stress can be the factor that switches it on. For example, Sieminski has depression, as does her mother. What she attributes her depression to, however, is a stressor: a childhood friend's death by suicide.

The stress teens experience comes from a variety of places. For Sieminski, it was a traumatic experience. The same goes for

US Olympic gymnast Simone Biles, who attributed her depression to sexual assault. For others, it might be academics, family dynamics, the COVID-19 pandemic, social media, or some other trigger.

Sieminski and Biles are not alone in facing depression in connection with trauma. Sunny, for example, had begun getting treatment for depression and anxiety when she was thirteen. Her mental health was improving, but that changed when her cousin died in a car crash. "That year started off as a wreck when he died in January. It was really tough that year. I struggled to keep my grades up and my anxiety/depression proceeded to get worse,"[30] she explains in a blog post. Steven "B" Smith succumbed to depression when he was sixteen, after his best friend accidentally shot him and he became unable to walk or breathe on his own. In B's case, not only did he have to face the trauma of being shot but also the trauma of suddenly becoming disabled. B was so depressed that he didn't want to do any of the therapy that would help him—although he later changed his mind, which also improved his mood.

Additionally, people who experience depression in the wake of trauma can experience post-traumatic stress disorder (PTSD). PTSD and depression not only can happen at the same time but also can have symptoms that overlap, such as problems sleeping or concentrating. In fact, people who have PTSD are up to five times more likely to have depression than those who do not have PTSD, according to the US Department of Veterans Affairs. Nonetheless, PTSD and depression are not the same thing. PTSD involves flashbacks, an exaggerated response to being startled, avoiding reminders of the traumatic experience, and being extraordinarily careful in avoiding trauma in the future. PTSD can lead to depression, but it is not depression.

Social Media Use

Although trauma is one stressor that can influence the incidence of depression, another stressor that teens face and can influence mental health is social media use. Platforms such as Instagram, Facebook, Snapchat, TikTok, and X (formerly Twitter) are now used by almost every US teen, according to the US Department of Health and Human Services. These platforms are increasingly being seen as a cause of depression in young people. In May 2023, Surgeon General Murthy issued a warning about social media use by children and teens. "There are ample indicators that social media can . . . have a profound risk of harm to the mental health and well-being of children and adolescents,"[31] Murthy stated in his report.

Social media use can cause young adolescent girls and boys to have less satisfaction with their lives because they feel like they are missing out on the fun experiences so many others seem to be posting about on social media platforms. Stress develops when teens compare themselves and their lives to the images and stories they see on social media. "A large part of the mental distress is around the pressure for perfection," says April Thames, a professor of psychiatry and a clinical neuropsychologist at the University of California, Los Angeles. "When you see people on these platforms constantly putting up in-your-face posts of their fabulous trips and beautiful filtered pictures, it creates a false standard for the youth, who are still trying to figure out their identity and where they fit in."[32]

The risks to mental health go beyond young social media users constantly comparing themselves to their peers. Social media has also become a vehicle for bullying. Recent scientific studies show that bullying online, which can spread widely and last forever, can lead to depression. Even negative comments that fall short of bullying can be bad. "Unfortunately, we tend to remember negative feedback more than we do positive, and on social media, those remarks linger where everybody can see them,"[33] explains Thames.

> "When you see people on these platforms constantly putting up in-your-face posts of their fabulous trips and beautiful filtered pictures, it creates a false standard for the youth, who are still trying to figure out their identity and where they fit in."[32]
>
> —April Thames, a professor of psychiatry and a clinical neuropsychologist at the University of California, Los Angeles

Some Say Social Media Use Can Help Alleviate Depression

Not all the news regarding social media use is bad. Some scientists say social media use can enhance mental health for some teens. It can do this by helping them connect with people who share their interests or experiences. This can be especially important for teens who feel alone or who lack connection with likeminded people in their communities. They can use social media to get emotional support from others.

Social media can benefit young people in other ways, too. For example, many teens use TikTok, Instagram, and other social media platforms to be creative and to express their ideas and talents. Social media platforms allow young people to see what is happening around the world, which can help them learn new things. Social media also allows teens, quite simply, to be entertained. "Social media that's humorous or distracting or provides a meaningful connection to peers and a wide social network might even help teens avoid depression," the Mayo Clinic states.

"Teens and Social Media Use: What's the Impact?," Mayo Clinic, February 26, 2022. www.mayoclinic.org.

Murthy cited various scientific studies in his report. Among them was a study that showed adolescents who spend more than three hours a day on social media may be at greater risk of mental health problems. That means virtually all adolescents are at risk because most spend at least that much time on those platforms daily.

COVID-19

Among other external factors that have led to higher rates of teen depression is the COVID-19 pandemic. The pandemic, which was declared a global health emergency in January 2020, dramatically changed daily life for nearly two years. Throughout the United States, schools, government buildings, and businesses were shut down to try to stem the spread of the virus. Students who were used to going to their school buildings each day had to take classes remotely using computers, so they no longer saw their friends and teachers. Extracurricular activities were suspended. After-school jobs disappeared. Shopping in stores and visiting extended family on the weekends and on holidays ended. Some students did not return to school in person until fall of 2021. Others went to schools with hybrid learning in which half the school population would go to school one day and the other half would attend school via computer, and then they would alternate the next day.

Once schools reopened in-person classes for all students, which for many was during the 2021–2022 school year, students told researchers they were more depressed and more anxious as a result of the changes caused by the pandemic. Another study showed youth depression doubled during the pandemic compared to the level reported prior to the pandemic. "The disruption to their routines and consistency is very damaging for a child's mental health," Jenna Glover, a child clinical psychologist and di-

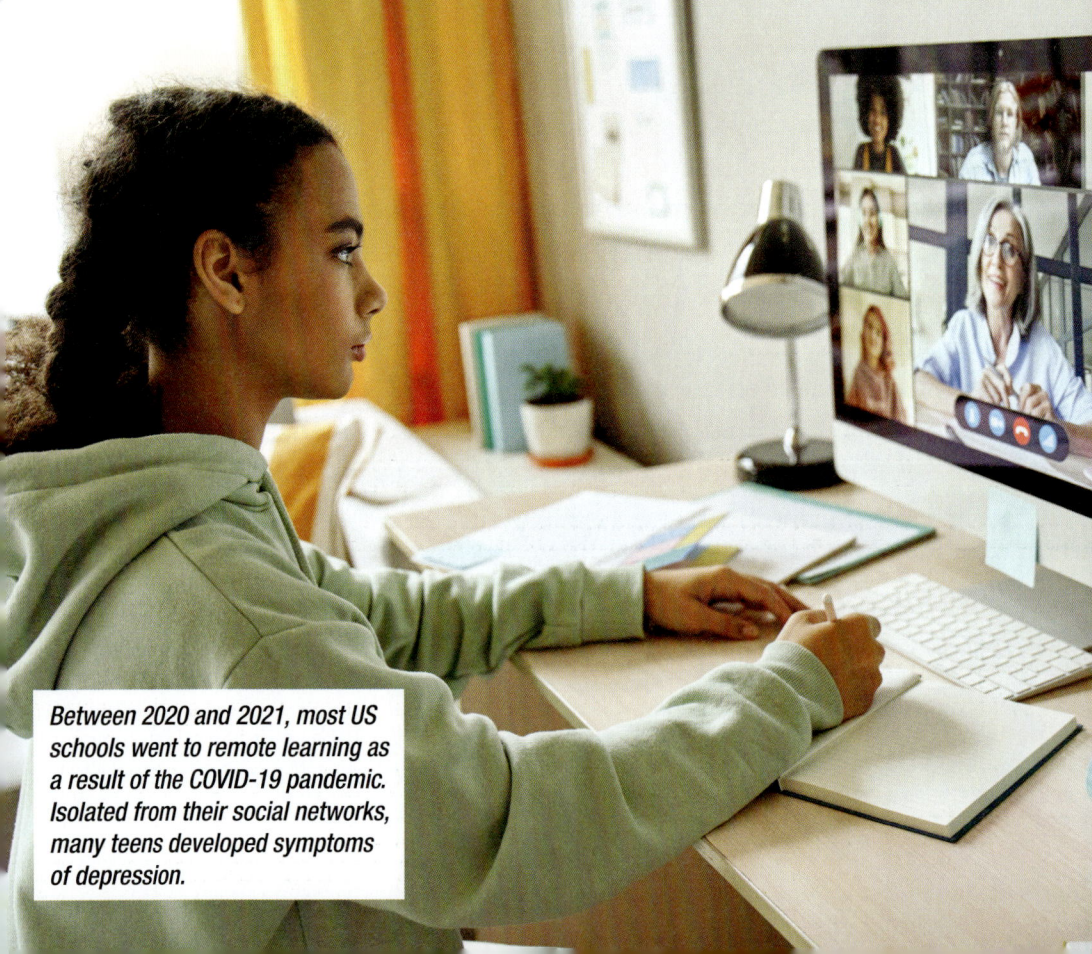

Between 2020 and 2021, most US schools went to remote learning as a result of the COVID-19 pandemic. Isolated from their social networks, many teens developed symptoms of depression.

rector of psychology training at Children's Hospital Colorado, said in 2021. "They thrive on predictability, which has been absent for over a year."[34]

Among those whose depression escalated during the pandemic was M. With no friends around, M pretended to go to virtual school but watched an anime series instead, then would feel bad about not doing the work. M labeled the cause of their mental health problems: "Loneliness."[35]

Clearly, no single factor can be labeled as a cause of depression. For one person, it could be surviving violence. For another, it could be experiencing a profound loss. For others, it could be social media use that negatively affects their confidence and feeling of safety. For still others, it could be built into their DNA. Because depression can be linked to more than one cause, relieving the symptoms of depression can be complicated and challenging, requiring trial and error.

CHAPTER FOUR

Getting Treatment

Help is available from mental health providers for teens with depression, but some young people cannot get that help. "Adolescents' families and caregivers must navigate various barriers to access behavioral health treatments for both outpatient and inpatient services," wrote Malini Ghoshal in a June 2022 article on the MedCentral website. "Obstacles may include familial, clinical, or socio-environmental considerations."[36] A clinical obstacle might be having little or no access to a professional office staffed with mental health providers. A socio-environmental obstacle might include not having the money to pay for mental health care or being a member of a cultural group that has less access to mental health care than others. A familial obstacle might be having family members who believe that seeking help with mental health is a sign of weakness or will bring unfavorable attention from outsiders.

Shame and stigma also can make adolescents reluctant to get help. In fact, according to the Mayo Clinic, getting help is a way to relieve the shame and stigma of having a mental illness. US gymnast Simone Biles, who revealed publicly that she became depressed in the wake of sexual assault, encouraged young people to seek the assistance they need anyway. "It's OK to say I need help and there's nothing wrong with that,"[37] she explains.

Once a person seeks treatment from a mental health professional, chances are very good for some, if not complete, relief from depressive symptoms. The APA says somewhere between 80 percent and 90 percent of people who seek treatment get good results.

Various medical treatments exist for adolescent depression, the most effective of which may be a combination of medication and talk therapy. The talk therapies recommended by the American Psychological Association include cognitive behavioral therapy (CBT) and interpersonal psychotherapy for adolescents. That combination is supported by science. "Cognitive behavioral therapy and another therapy, interpersonal therapy, have the most evidence for treating adolescent depression,"[38] report doctors Ana Radovic and Megan A. Moreno.

> "It's OK to say I need help and there's nothing wrong with that."[37]
>
> —Simone Biles, an Olympic gymnast who experienced depression because of sexual assault

Psychotherapy

Psychotherapy is talk therapy. It is conducted by a mental health professional. This could be a counselor, social worker, psychologist, or psychiatrist. The professional and the person seeking treatment typically meet weekly or biweekly for hourly sessions. The meetings can be in person at the therapist's office or via online meeting technology, such as Zoom or Google Meets. During therapy sessions, patients talk about their emotions, behavior, and experiences while the mental health provider helps the individual find healthy ways to cope with the illness.

Among well-known young people who have undergone therapy for depression is actor Zendaya. She gained fame as a young teen when she starred in *Shake It Up* on the Disney Channel and later went on to star in HBO's *Euphoria*. "There's nothing wrong with working on yourself and dealing with those things with someone who can help you, someone who can talk to you, who's not your mom or whatever, who has no bias,"[39] Zendaya said in 2021.

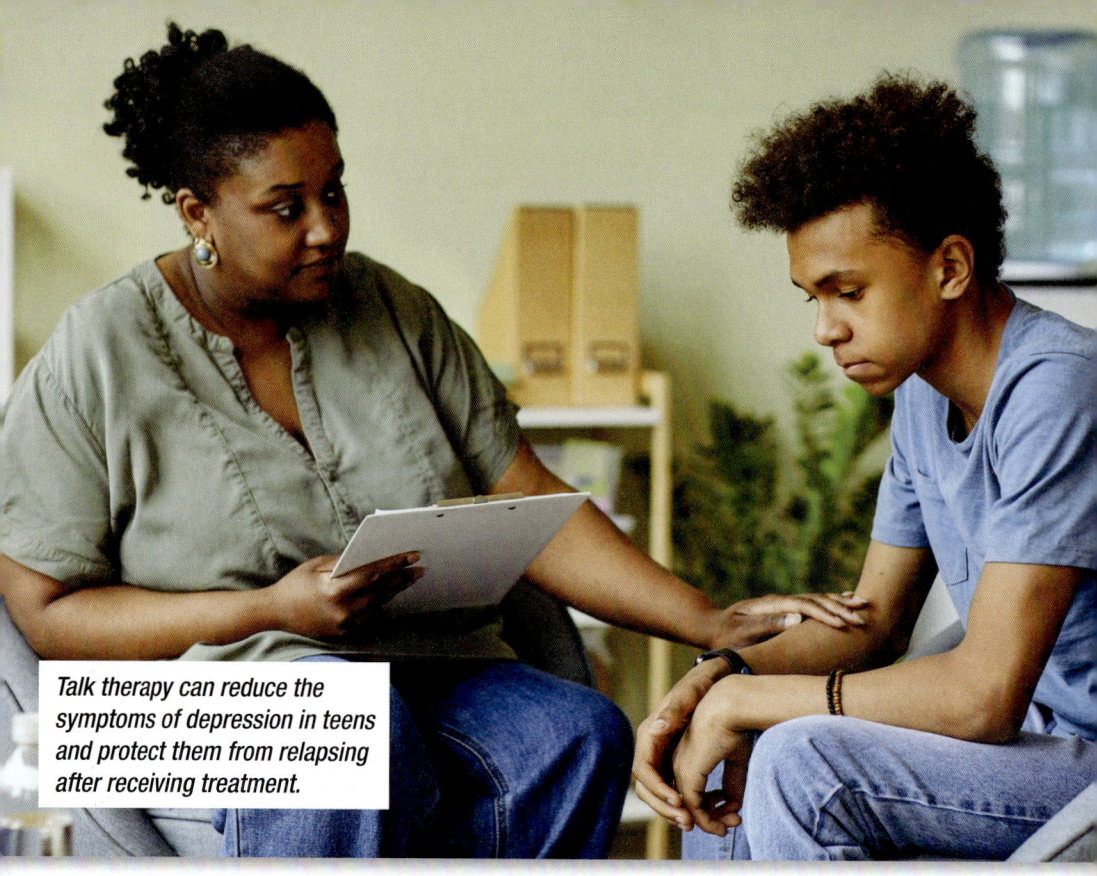

Talk therapy can reduce the symptoms of depression in teens and protect them from relapsing after receiving treatment.

    One type of psychotherapy for teens with depression is CBT. It's a type of talk therapy in which the mental health provider listens to the depressed person talk about his or her thoughts and emotions and then guides the person to recognize how those thoughts may be overly negative or not based on fact. Here's an example of an irrational thought: "I'm a complete failure. I mess up everything, and that's why everyone hates me." After the depressed teen becomes aware of the irrational thoughts, the therapist's job is to help the teen change that thinking and learn to think and respond to those irrational thoughts in a healthier way. Therapists, who typically see patients over the course of five to twenty weeks, help their patients with coping, relationship, and problem-solving skills. Research indicates that CBT works. A study by Dutch researchers that was published in 2019 by the Cambridge University Press concluded that CBT reduced the symptoms of depression in teens and protected them from relapsing after receiving treatment.

The second type of therapy recommended for teens by the American Psychological Association is interpersonal psychotherapy. This therapy focuses exclusively on how the patient's relationships with other people are connected to the patient's depression. This therapy usually involves weekly hour-long sessions that take place over the course of three to four months.

In early sessions of interpersonal therapy, the teen lists important relationships and the strengths and challenges with each. After that, together with the therapist, the teen figures out which of the relationships is contributing to the teen's depression. During those early sessions, the teen and the therapist also create a statement of the goals of treatment. Later, the therapist works to help the teen develop, learn, and practice new ways to approach that relationship and figure out other ways to solve relationship challenges. Research shows that interpersonal therapy works for mild to moderate adolescent depression.

The Stigma Surrounding Depression

One reason some people hesitate to get help for depression is because they are afraid of what other people will think about them having a mental illness.

Stigma stems from fear. When people do not understand something, like why a person is behaving unusually, they may become afraid of it. Centuries ago, before people knew that mental illness was a medical problem, many societies thought people with such illnesses were possessed by evil spirits or the devil. As a result, people who were experiencing mental illness were killed, subjected to torturous medical treatments, or locked up.

Nowadays, the climate surrounding mental health treatment has improved, perhaps because well-known people like Lady Gaga and Justin Bieber have spoken about having depression. Still, more change is needed.

Among the ways to change attitudes is to look at mental illness as a physical illness, because that's what it is. The brain is part of the physical person, just the way a heart or spleen is. Also, be aware of the language used to describe those with mental illness, and speak in a way that shows the disease is not the person. Don't refer to "the mentally ill"; refer instead to "people with mental illnesses."

Medication

Psychotherapy alone reduces symptoms of depression in some young people. Others have better results from a combination of therapy and medication. Still others find medication alone will do the trick. Some well-known entertainers, such as singer Katy Perry, have stated publicly that they have taken antidepressant medication. "It was one of those things where I'd sprained my brain a little bit," Perry said. "I felt like I needed crutches for my brain, and I did. And I used those crutches to get back on my feet."[40] For those who need medication for their depressive symptoms, a variety are available. Medications should only be used after consulting with a medical doctor such as a primary care physician or a psychiatrist.

There are a variety of medications used to help teens manage depression. The broad term for these medications is *antidepressants*. Selective serotonin reuptake inhibitors (SSRIs) are the medications prescribed most often to combat adolescent depression. That's because in addition to being effective, SSRIs tend to have fewer side effects than other classes of drugs prescribed for depression. SSRIs work by increasing the amount of serotonin in the brain. Serotonin is a chemical known as a neurotransmitter. It has many jobs, including controlling moods.

> "I felt like I needed crutches for my brain, and I did. And I used those crutches to get back on my feet."[40]
>
> —Katy Perry, a singer who has taken antidepressant medication

As levels of serotonin increase, feelings of depression decrease. Sometimes such drugs are all that's needed for depression relief. At other times, because the medication has reduced a person's depressive symptoms, they are able to participate in other treatment that may be required, such as talk therapy.

A number of different SSRIs are on the market. Fluoxetine, better known as Prozac, is the drug most often prescribed to teens with depression, perhaps because it is the SSRI that's been most studied by scientists and proven effective in young people.

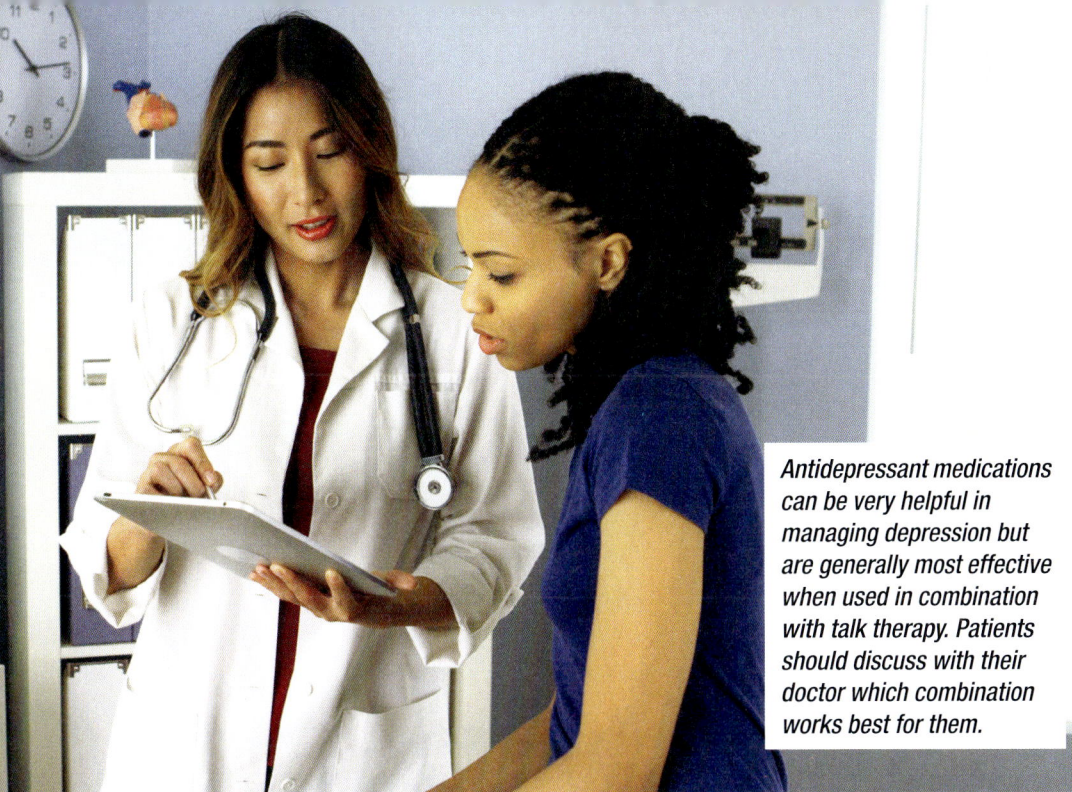

Antidepressant medications can be very helpful in managing depression but are generally most effective when used in combination with talk therapy. Patients should discuss with their doctor which combination works best for them.

SSRIs do not work for everyone, however. Another type of medication used for managing depression in teens is known as a serotonin-norepinephrine reuptake inhibitor (SNRI). These drugs boost the levels of both serotonin and norepinephrine. Whereas serotonin regulates moods, norepinephrine regulates attention, thinking, and reaction to stress. Because SNRIs affect two brain chemicals rather than one, they tend to have more side effects. That's why doctors prescribe SSRIs as the first course of action for teens who need help managing depression. Doctors have a variety of other drugs they can prescribe for teens if SSRIs and SNRIs do not achieve desired results. These other drugs tend to have more serious side effects, so they are used less often for teens with depression.

Medication Drawbacks

Side effects are the main drawbacks of taking medication. Most side effects are mild and go away after the body gets used to the drug. Among the possible side effects for SSRIs, for example,

How to Find a Therapist

The first step in getting help for depression is recognizing the problem exists. After that comes finding a therapist. One way to do that is to ask family, friends, the family doctor, or even a school guidance counselor for references. If your family has health insurance, the insurance company might also have a list of preferred therapists.

Getting a list of therapists is the easy part. The harder part is finding one that makes the patient feel comfortable and provides the sort of therapy that will work for that person. That may require phone interviews as well as in-person interviews. Sometimes a patient will need to visit several different therapists before finding the right one.

Finding the right therapist is of paramount importance because that person will play a pivotal role in restoring mental health to the young patient. "Your relationship with your therapist has more impact on outcomes than the techniques used," comments psychologist Andrew Damian. "This is likely because no technique will work, no matter how advanced it is, if you don't feel safe or trust your therapist."

Andrew Damian, "What Influences Successful Psychotherapy?," Mind-Body Treatment, March 31, 2020. www.mindbodytreatment.com.

---

are nausea, headaches, and sleepiness. Antidepressants can also interfere with rapid eye movement (REM) sleep. REM sleep is thought to be important in mood regulation. Some stronger antidepressant drugs prescribed for teens have worse side effects, including a sudden rise in blood pressure that could be deadly. These stronger drugs are used only when other drugs fail to provide relief to teens suffering from depression.

People also can experience side effects—withdrawal-type symptoms and a worsening of depression—if they suddenly stop taking antidepressants. Patients must consult with their doctors if they want to stop taking their medication, and their doctors will come up with a plan to gradually wean them off the medication.

In addition, the federal government requires drug companies to put a warning label on the antidepressants they manufacture. That warning label states that the use of those drugs may lead to suicidal thoughts in young people. The government requires the warning because when it reviewed clinical trials of antidepressant use in young people, it found that a small number of those taking the drugs had an increase in suicidal thoughts.

Scientists do not know why those suicidal thoughts increase in some young people. Research thus far does not show that taking antidepressants causes people to die by suicide, according to the Mayo Clinic. None of the young people in those trials acted on the suicidal thoughts linked to antidepressant use. Research also exists that shows suicide rates go down when teens take antidepressants.

Brain Stimulation Therapy

Although many medications are available, sometimes they do not work. When that happens, and the teen has severe depression, doctors may recommend that electric current be used to impact the neurotransmitters in the patient's brain. This is called brain stimulation therapy.

One type of brain stimulation therapy is electroconvulsive therapy (ECT), which is approved for use in teens. The patient is given general anesthesia—so the person is unconscious for the procedure—and a muscle-relaxing medication. Electrodes are placed on the patient's head, and an electrical current is sent into the brain to cause a seizure that affects the neurotransmitters. The seizure lasts less than a minute, and the patient wakes in five to ten minutes. ECT is typically administered three times a week for six to twelve weeks. Usually those who undergo the therapy must take antidepressants after the treatment period to maintain the improvement in symptoms and ensure they don't come back. Sometimes patients need to get ECT periodically to maintain progress against depression.

Hannah's Story

Beginning when she was a young teen, Hannah Wyatt Sultan began experiencing mental illnesses. Among the mental illnesses was depression, which set in when she was in college and in an abusive relationship. Depression caused her to take a break from college at one point and then, later, not one but two breaks from nursing studies. She used prescribed medications to treat her illness, but the medicine stopped working.

While in nursing school, Hannah had heard about ECT and eventually sought that treatment. She received outpatient ECT for about ten weeks and started feeling better after the first week. "It was shocking—pun intended—how well it worked," she says. "I was feeling dramatically better after my second treatment."[41]

After ECT, Hannah and her doctor created an exercise and psychotherapy plan designed to help her maintain her mental health. "It's like the mind is a garden with tons of weeds," explains Dr. Konoy Mandal, who administered ECT to Hannah. "ECT clears the weeds, it tills, it brings the water and all of that, but it doesn't plant anything. ECT is only as good as the therapy that follows it. That's where patients make enduring changes in their brain."[42]

Like antidepressants, brain stimulation therapies have a range of side effects. For ECT, some patients experience headaches, muscle aches, memory loss, upset stomach, and disorientation. Hannah experienced temporary short-term memory loss.

Hospital and Residential Treatment

With most treatments for depression, young patients live at home and regularly attend school. However, sometimes those with depression are so ill that they cannot take care of themselves properly or they may be in danger of hurting themselves or other people. In such cases, patients may need to stay in a hospital or move into a psychiatric treatment center to get round-the-clock treatment and stay safe.

The number of such hospitalizations has been rising. Pediatric mental health hospitalizations increased to almost 202,000 in 2019—a jump of almost 26 percent from 2009—according to a March 2023 article in the *Journal of the American Medical Association*.

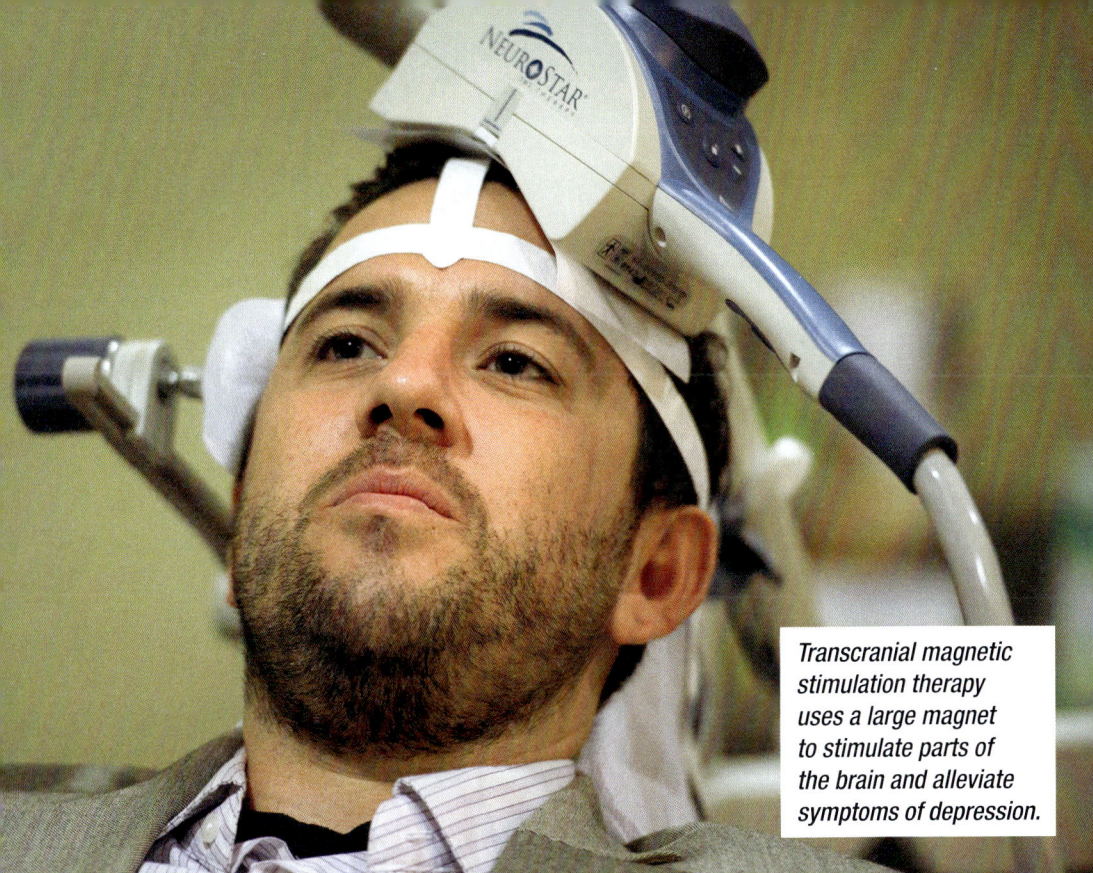

Transcranial magnetic stimulation therapy uses a large magnet to stimulate parts of the brain and alleviate symptoms of depression.

Among those who spent time in an in-patient psychiatric facility was Sophia Juhas, who had anxiety and depression most of her life. As she became older, her illness worsened. When she was in her midteens, Sophia was thinking about dying by suicide. That prompted a six-day stay at the Behavioral Health Center at Children's Hospital New Orleans in January 2022. "We specifically worked on a lot of coping strategies because dealing with anxiety was sort of new to me," Sophia explains.

> I had developed my own coping skills but not the ones that were proven to work. I met people with anxiety disorders and depression who were just like me, and people with more severe diagnoses. We worked in small and large groups. We did music therapy and art therapy together. The nurses and staff made me feel comfortable as I could be in the hospital. I also made new friends there.[43]

Once Sophia left the hospital, however, the stress of daily life brought a return of depressive symptoms. This prompted a second hospitalization. "By the time I left the hospital for the second time, I felt empowered," Sophia says. "I could see a bright future ahead of me."[44]

Finding the Right Treatment Requires Patience

The treatments offered by mental health providers to teens with depression are extensive and varied. Finding the right treatment often requires patience. It is not unusual to have to try more than one treatment before finding the best solution. However, research shows that young people experiencing depression often respond well to those treatments. "Depression in children and adolescents can be safely and effectively treated," wrote C. Scott Moreland and Liza Bonin in an October 3, 2022, article published by UpToDate, a subscription-based website that provides clinical information to doctors. "Psychological treatments (psychotherapy), medication therapy (pharmacotherapy), and other measures can alleviate symptoms and help children and adolescents to succeed in school, develop and maintain healthy relationships, and feel more self-confident."[45]

CHAPTER FIVE

Lifestyle Changes Can Help Fight Depression

In fourth grade, Skylar Moore began experiencing depression when it occurred to her that people are judged for the way they look, and she did not think she was pretty. By the time Skylar reached high school, depression led her to believe that not only her appearance but also nearly everything about her was wrong. It made her angry, irritable, and constantly sad. "Depression's like being trapped and seeing the light—seeing the end—and not knowing how to get it,"[46] Skylar explains. With professional help that included psychotherapy and antidepressant medications, Skylar's symptoms improved, and the girl who had no friends as a high school freshman found herself on the homecoming court as a senior.

Seeking professional help, as Skylar did with the urging of her mother, is a big step toward coping with depression. Teens have other steps they can take as well. Teens who experience depression or are at risk of developing it can take some steps on their own to maintain mental health. These actions are called protective factors, and they are things people should do to keep their bodies—including their brains—healthy. Protective factors include eating healthfully, getting the proper amount and quality of sleep, and exercising.

Diet

One area of particular interest for researchers is diet. Researchers who analyzed scientific studies that focused on what people with depression eat found that a healthy diet was associated with a lower risk of developing depression. A healthy diet includes fruits, vegetables, nuts, fish, and whole grains. Conversely, eating a diet full of red meat, refined grains like white flour, high-fat foods like cheese and butter, and sweets is associated with an increased risk of developing depression.

For Jane Green, who was diagnosed with depression when she was fourteen, changing her diet to reduce sugar intake went a long way to changing her mental health for the better. Jane went to therapy and took prescribed antidepressant medication, but her symptoms remained until she ditched her habit of eating candy and ice cream every day and instead began eating more vegetables, healthy fats, and protein. "I wasn't focusing on what I couldn't eat—I was focusing on how great I felt physically, which made me feel better mentally and emotionally," Jane says. "I stopped getting the crazy highs and lows from sugar."[47] In fact, depressive symptoms decreased to such a degree that Jane no longer needed antidepressants.

Catherine Hayes tells a story similar to Green's. Catherine suffered with depressive symptoms that included mood swings, low self-esteem, and even a desire to die. At the time, Catherine's diet included daily sweets, such as cookies in the afternoon with coffee and dessert after dinner.

Catherine changed her diet after looking into other ways she could cope with depression in addition to taking antidepressant medications. Her new diet included a lot of greens and other vegetables as well as healthy fats and proteins, and it reduced sugar intake by ditching sweet salad dressings for oil and lemon juice and eating low-sugar fresh fruits such as blueberries. "My energy levels picked up," Catherine recalls. "I was finally sleeping. My moods weren't as low. I was happier, and the anxiety and depression just didn't seem to be there."[48] Like Jane, Catherine was able

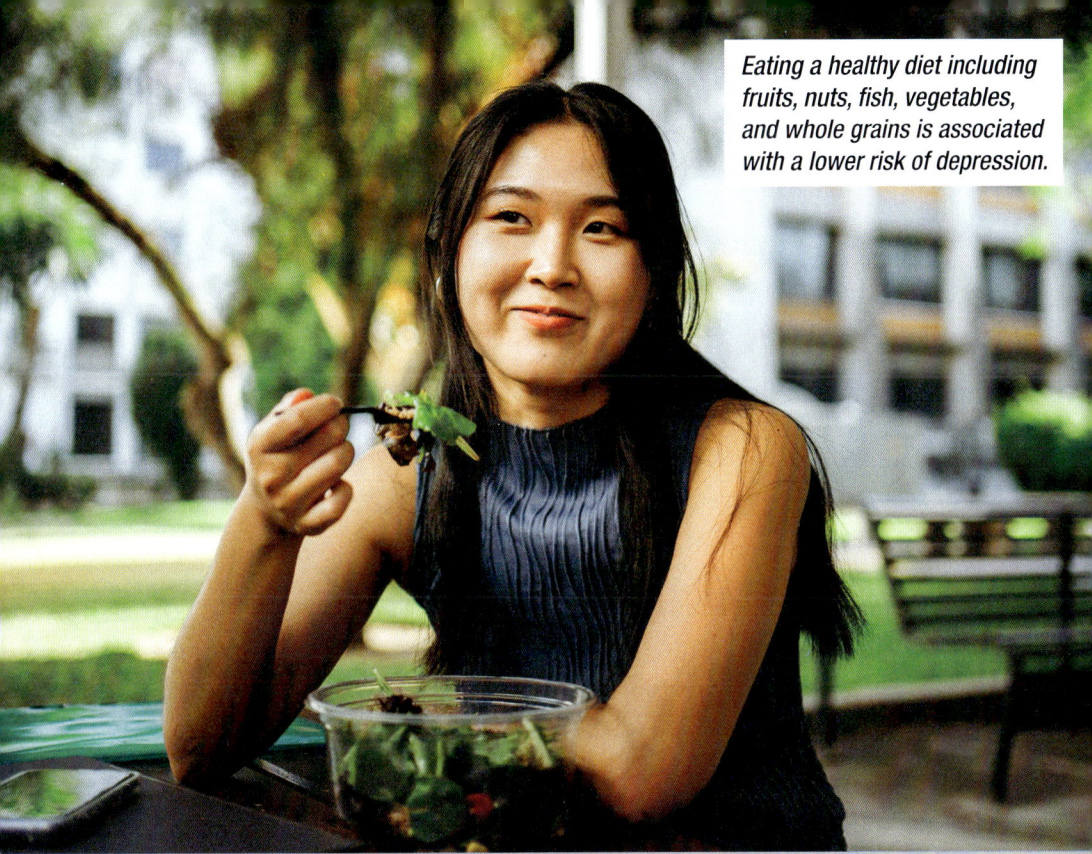

Eating a healthy diet including fruits, nuts, fish, vegetables, and whole grains is associated with a lower risk of depression.

to gradually stop taking antidepressant medication—something that should only be done under a doctor's care.

Several factors may be at play regarding the effect of diet on depression. Regarding sugar intake, a 2019 study published in the journal *Neuroscience & Biobehavioral Reviews* found a link between a high-sugar diet and depression. The study said eating too much sugar may alter the way a person perceives and processes emotion. Regarding eating vitamin-rich vegetables, science has shown that vitamins help with the creation of serotonin, a brain chemical that plays a role in feeling the emotion of happiness.

Nonetheless, teens who are depressed should seek professional mental health care first and try dietary changes to support whatever other medical interventions the teen, the teen's family, and the teen's doctor agree to try. "I'm all in favor of helping people take a look at their fitness and diet as a holistic plan to help recover from depression, but I wouldn't count on it solely,"[49] advises Michael Thase, a psychiatrist at the University of Pennsylvania.

Meditation

Some experts recommend meditation to reduce stress, anxiety, and depression. Done properly, meditation can help people focus on the moment rather than think about bad things that happened in the past or worry about bad things that might happen in the future. This can relieve depressive symptoms by training the brain not to get stuck on negative thoughts.

To meditate, a person should sit in a quiet place and pay attention to their breath going in and out. When first starting to practice meditation, most people find that they begin by focusing on their breathing, but then their minds quickly wander to thinking about the past or future. The idea is to practice refocusing on your breath. Start out doing this for five minutes a day. With practice, it becomes easier to focus on breathing only and not on anything else.

Experts say meditation may help reduce depressive symptoms. It also has other benefits, including reducing stress, increasing focus, reducing anxiety, improving sleep, and improving willpower.

Sleep

In addition to eating well, people should get a good night's sleep to help ward off depression. Poor sleep is a risk factor for depression. A 2019 study conducted by Rachel Widome of the University of Minnesota showed that about 33 percent of high school students who slept less than six hours per night had a high number of depression symptoms; in contrast, about 10 percent of those who got adequate sleep had a high number of depression symptoms. "Poor sleep and depression are reinforcing—depression interferes with sleep, and not enough sleep leaves someone feeling like they don't have energy to engage in life, which is a symptom of depression,"[50] Widome explains.

That is what happened to Ben Freedman, who was seventeen and a high school junior when he became depressed. "I was way tired out," says Ben, who reported getting five to six hours of sleep each night, although his father said Ben was sleeping less than that. "And less sleep put me in a really, really depressed state. I was suffering really badly."[51] Ben committed to getting more sleep to help resolve his depression. He also participated in psychotherapy and took prescribed antidepressants.

Experts say teens should sleep eight to ten hours a day. This can be difficult for young people who not only go to school but also participate in extracurricular activities, have responsibilities at home, and have jobs. To get a good night's sleep, adolescents should stick to a regular sleep schedule that includes avoiding sleeping in on the weekends. They also should cut down on television and phone use at night because the light from the devices can confuse the body and interfere with the natural sleep-wake cycle. Avoiding caffeine before bed can help. Meditation can help improve sleep too, as can exercise.

Exercise

Not only can exercise help improve sleep, it also is a protective factor against developing depressive symptoms. People with higher levels of physical activity are less likely to have the symptoms of depression. Conversely, people with lower levels of physical activity—less than the recommended 150 minutes of moderate to vigorous exercise each week—are more likely to have depression.

Exercise is what helped Marci Goldberg, who was diagnosed with depression and anxiety when she was in high school. She began competing in triathlons, in which participants swim, run, and bicycle. Triathlon training became her most important tool for managing her mental health. "I have those days that something happened the day before or moments before and I just don't want to get my training in," Goldberg writes in a blog post. "Those are the days I have to tell myself that I am capable of so much. It's really in times like these that I tell myself I'm training to help my mental health over training for races."[52]

> "I tell myself I'm training to help my mental health over training for races."[52]
>
> —Marci Goldberg, who participates in triathlons to help her depression

In addition to managing stress, making a person physically stronger, and helping with relaxation, exercise also builds self-esteem, which is something that suffers when a person is depressed. People with depression may feel tired and may not feel like doing anything. Not doing anything can make the person feel

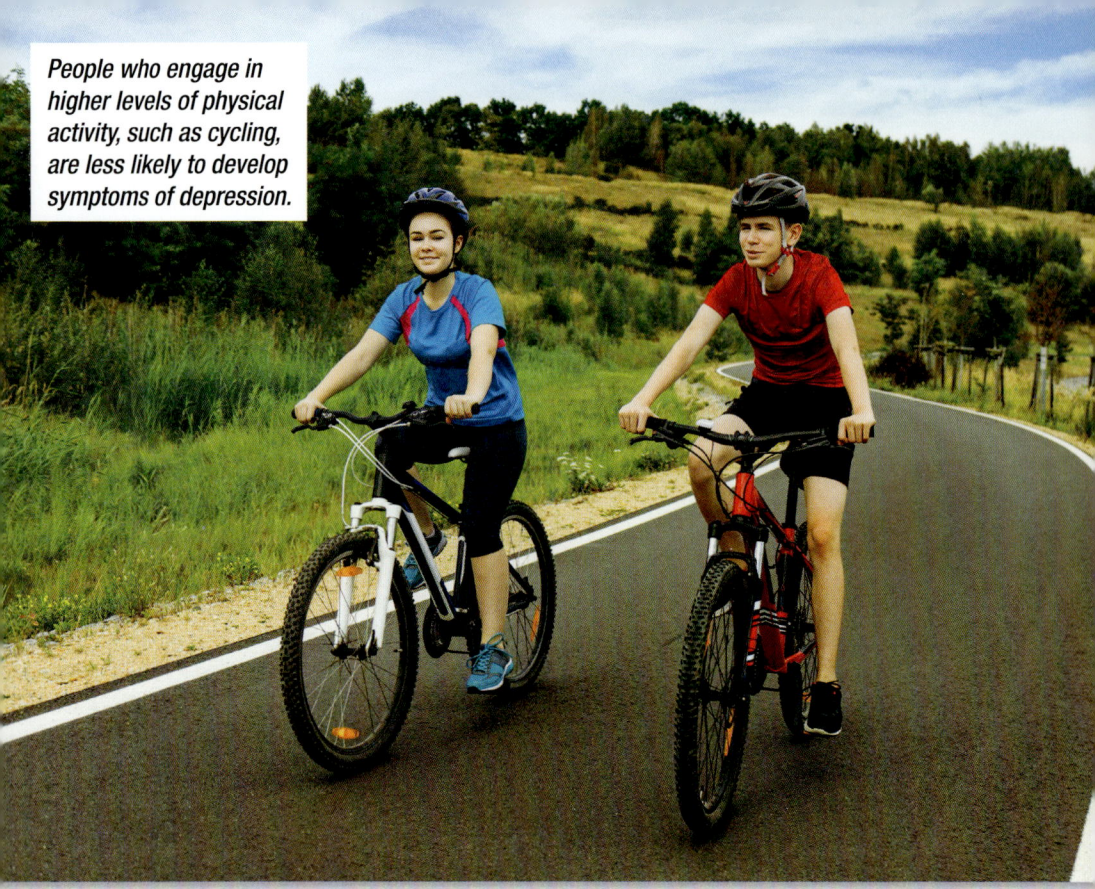

People who engage in higher levels of physical activity, such as cycling, are less likely to develop symptoms of depression.

guilty or lazy or a failure, which can make the person lose self-esteem. Exercise can help a person combat those feelings of laziness or failure. "Exercising also gives someone a sense of accomplishment, another reason why it can help with depression,"[53] explains Dr. Danielle Hairston, a psychiatrist.

Social Connection

Joining a sports team, taking a dance class or exercise class, finding a walking or hiking group, or doing something active with others offers additional help in the fight against depression. First, it increases physical activity; second, it offers opportunities for socializing. Socializing keeps people from isolating themselves and focusing on negative thoughts. In 2020, researchers from Massachusetts General Hospital (MGH) determined that having positive relationships with others was the strongest protective factor against becoming depressed. "Far and away the most prominent of these [protective] factors was frequency of confiding in others, but also visits with family and friends, all of which highlighted the important protective effect of social connection and social cohesion,"[54] states Jordan Smoller, a psychiatrist and the senior author of the study.

Scientific studies have examined this issue. The connections teens had with family and friends were a main influence on whether the teens described themselves as depressed or not, according to a January 2021 study. Meeting people and making friends can boost self-esteem. Researchers found that positive, healthy relationships help create and improve self-esteem in people of all ages, teens included. Having positive relationships also helps a person with depression to have support when things are not going well.

> "Far and away the most prominent of these [protective] factors was frequency of confiding in others, but also visits with family and friends, all of which highlighted the important protective effect of social connection and social cohesion."[54]
>
> —Jordan Smoller, psychiatrist

Reducing Stress

Besides getting a good night's sleep, eating healthy food, exercising, and socializing, reducing stress also can protect against depression. The body's reaction to stress impacts brain chemistry, and being under stress for a long time can lead to depression. "Our stress response does pretty good in the short term, but it doesn't do very good if you activate it in the long term," states David Prescott, an associate professor of health administration and public health. "If we stay under chronic stress, our physiological stress response is taxed beyond what it's designed to do, and it starts to impair us."[55]

People can manage stress in a variety of ways, among which are listening to music, exercising, meditation, and yoga. Meditation offers a way for people to train themselves to shift their thinking away from negative thoughts and emotions, producing relaxation and calm. Yoga involves physical poses, breathing exercises, and meditation, which together reduce stress and improve overall health.

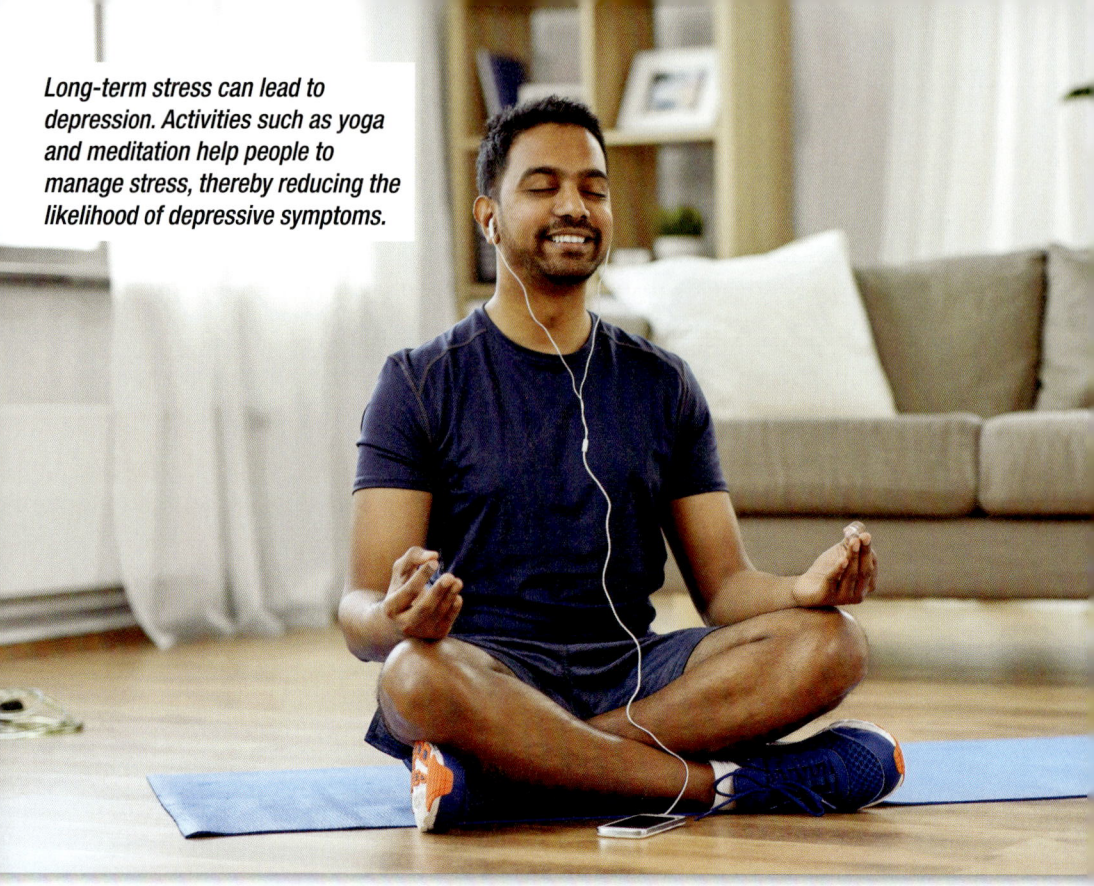

Long-term stress can lead to depression. Activities such as yoga and meditation help people to manage stress, thereby reducing the likelihood of depressive symptoms.

Stay Away from Alcohol and Recreational Drugs

Staying away from drugs and alcohol is another way to prevent and reduce depression. Alcohol is a depressant that slows down brain activity. While it lowers anxiety, stress, and fear, it also lowers norepinephrine and serotonin, two of the brain chemicals that regulate mood. Although people often say they drink alcohol to make themselves feel better, alcohol actually worsens depression. People with depression who drink too much will have more and worse bouts of depression. Additionally, they may wind up with a second problem—alcoholism—on top of their depression.

That is what happened to James Dawson, who had depression and anxiety. His depression led him to drink alcohol daily, beginning when he was a teen. James's drinking led to alcohol dependence rather than a cure for depression. "I realized my alcoholism was rooted in a deep-seated mental health issue that I had carried most of my life," James writes in a blog post. "Once the alcohol was out of the way, I was able to focus solely on my mental health."[56]

Alcoholism is not the only problem that can be caused when depressed people use alcohol. Alcohol interferes with the effectiveness of antidepressants. Alcohol also disrupts sleep, which is bad for mood regulation. Furthermore, drinking interferes with thinking. Making a bad decision while drinking—a decision that a person would not make while sober—can lead to bad consequences that make a person depressed.

As is the case with alcohol, some drugs, such as heroin and Xanax, are depressants and can lead to depression. Others, such as cocaine, Ecstasy, and meth, are stimulants. Stimulants can interfere with mood regulation too. Cannabis, or marijuana, can be classified as a depressant and a stimulant. Drugs like these change the way the brain works, and that can lead to or worsen depression. For example, a 2023 study by Columbia University concluded that teens who use cannabis recreationally—in other words, teens who do not have a cannabis dependency—are two to four times more likely to develop depression and other psychiatric disorders than teens who do not use cannabis.

How to Support Others Who Have Depression

Knowing the symptoms of depression will not only help people recognize that they are having a problem but also help them recognize that a friend or family member may be depressed. If loved ones or friends stop enjoying things they used to love, or they stay home alone a lot when they used to hang out with others, it may be time to step up and help.

Helping involves talking to the person about the changes in their mood and behavior and why that is a worry. Sometimes people self-stigmatize—they think they're weak or weird if they can't stop thinking negative thoughts. They may need to hear that problems with the brain are no more a result of a personal flaw than any other illness.

Encourage the friend or loved one to go to a family doctor or a mental health provider to assess the situation. Even offer to look for doctors or other professionals, make appointments, and arrange travel if that is what it takes to make sure the person gets the needed help.

In addition, those who are depressed are more likely to develop a substance use disorder if they turn to drugs to relieve the symptoms of depression. If the substances provide some relief, that may encourage depressed people to use them more, which can lead to dependence.

The Good News

Staying away from unhealthy behaviors like using drugs and drinking and eating unhealthy food may also ward off the mental illness altogether. Embracing healthy behaviors like eating nourishing food, exercising, getting a good night's sleep, reducing stress, and maintaining positive connections with others can do the same thing. However, if depression occurs, people have a lot of tools they can use to get relief. First, they have to recognize the symptoms and seek help from mental health providers. After that, they should take their prescribed medication and go to therapy. Furthermore, they should make positive lifestyle changes, like exercising, eating right, sleeping well, reducing stress, and connecting with others. In fact, by following their treatment plans, a vast majority of people with depression will see their mental health improve.

That is what happened for Jack Bliss, who struggled with depression in high school. He urged others to get help, like he did. "If your symptoms are like mine, it probably won't feel like it can get better, but if you let your family or counselor or therapist or doctor try to help you, they probably can help," Bliss says. "The first thing might not work, but let them try anyway. And if you don't believe that you can get better, tell your depressed self to pretend that it can get better, and let people help you because it makes them feel better. That can be enough. Just hold on."[57]

SOURCE NOTES

Introduction: When Depression Strikes Teens

1. Quoted in Matt Richtel, "'It's Life or Death': The Mental Health Crisis Among U.S. Teens," *New York Times,* May 3, 2022. https://www.nytimes.com.
2. Quoted in Richtel, "'It's Life or Death.'"
3. Jamie Factor, "Writing Saved Me," Anxiety & Depression Association of America, June 24, 2023. https://adaa.org.
4. Factor, "Writing Saved Me."
5. Factor, "Writing Saved Me."
6. Madison Jo Sieminski, "Open Doors," Anxiety & Depression Association of America, February 25, 2020. https://adaa.org.
7. Sieminski, "Open Doors."

Chapter One: What Is Depression?

8. Sandra Mullen, "Major Depressive Disorder in Children and Adolescents," *Mental Health Clinician*, vol. 8, no. 6, November 2018. www.ncbi.nlm.nih.gov.
9. Mullen, "Major Depressive Disorder in Children and Adolescents."
10. Meg McCarney, "Meg McCarney Addresses Seasonal Affective Disorder," This Is My Brave, 2022. https://thisismybrave.org.
11. Quoted in Beverly Ford, "Owen's Struggles with Mental Health Didn't Hold Him Back—They Propelled Him Forward," *Boston Globe*, March 7, 2018. https://sponsored.bostonglobe.com.
12. Kimberly Zapata, "I Was a Teen with Depression—Here's What I Wish I Knew," *Parents*, May 4, 2023. www.parents.com.
13. New York University, Rory Meyers College of Nursing, "Depression May Look Different in Black Women," Press release, December 13, 2022. www.nyu.edu.

Chapter Two: Who Gets Depression?

14. Quoted in Office of the Surgeon General, *Protecting Youth Mental Health: The U.S. Surgeon General's Advisory*. Washington, DC: Office of the Surgeon General, US Department of Health and Human Services, 2021. www.hhs.gov.

15. Sylia Wilson and Nathalie M. Dumornay, "Rising Rates of Adolescent Depression in the United States: Challenges and Opportunities in the 2020s," *Journal of Adolescent Health,* vol. 70, no. 3, March 2022. www.jahonline.org.
16. Derek Thompson, "Why American Teens Are So Sad," *The Atlantic*, April 11, 2022. www.theatlantic.com.
17. Justin Bieber (@justinbieber), "It's hard to get out of bed in the morning when you are overwhelmed with your life, your past, job, responsibilities, emotions, your family, finances, your relationships," Instagram, September 2, 2019. www.instagram.com/p/B17JfkkHEKt/.
18. Justin Bieber, *Justin Bieber: The Next Chapter*, YouTube documentary, October 30, 2020. https://www.youtube.com/watch?v=RUcLuQ17UV8.
19. Quoted in Jason Bateman et al., "Billie Eilish & Finneas O'Connell," *Smartless* (podcast), February 15, 2021. https://podcasts.apple.com.
20. Quoted in Josh Eels, "Billie Eilish and the Triumph of the Weird," *Rolling Stone,* July 31, 2019. www.rollingstone.com.
21. Quoted in Lauren Valenti, "5 Young Celebrities Who Have Opened Up About Their Mental Health in 2019," *Vogue*, May 30, 2019. www.vogue.com.
22. Quoted in Erin Jensen, "Sophie Turner on Battle with Depression, Trolls and How Joe Jonas Helped Her Love Herself," *USA Today,* April 17, 2019. www.usatoday.com.
23. Simone Biles, "What More Can I Say?," *Simone vs. Herself*, Facebook Watch, July 6, 2021. www.facebook.com.
24. Quoted in Kerry Breen, "Lady Gaga's Mom Tells Sheinelle About Raising a Superstar, Bullying and Kindness," *Today*, January 27, 2020. www.today.com.
25. Quoted in Justin Moran, "Lady Gaga: Life on Chromatica," *Paper*, March 16, 2020. www.papermag.com.
26. Franciscan Children's, "A Survivor's Story: 7 Things I Learned from Teen Depression," *Boston*, November 2, 2017. www.bostonmagazine.com.

Chapter Three: Why Are Teens Depressed?

27. Sieminski, "Open Doors."
28. Jack Bliss, "Holding On: A Story About Teenage Depression," Community Child Guidance Clinic. www.ccgcinc.org.
29. Quoted in Lisa Bain and Hannah Jeon, "What 22 Celebrities Have Said About Having Depression, in Their Own Words," *Good Housekeeping*, February 3, 2020. www.goodhousekeeping.com.

30. Sunny, "A Teen's Story," Anxiety & Depression Association of America, December 12, 2022. https://adaa.org.
31. Quoted in Office of the Surgeon General, *Social Media and Youth Mental Health: The U.S. Surgeon General's Advisory.* Washington, DC: Office of the Surgeon General, US Department of Health and Human Services, 2023. www.hhs.gov.
32. Quoted in Chayil Champion, "Is Social Media Causing Psychological Harm to Youth and Young Adults?," UCLA Health, January 18, 2023. www.uclahealth.org.
33. Quoted in Champion, "Is Social Media Causing Psychological Harm to Youth and Young Adults?"
34. Quoted in Sarah Molano, "Youth Depression and Anxiety Doubled During the Pandemic, New Analysis Finds," CNN, August 10, 2021. www.cnn.com.
35. Quoted in Richtel, "'It's Life or Death.'"

Chapter Four: Getting Treatment

36. Malini Ghoshal, "Barriers and Challenges Impacting Adolescent Mental Health Treatment," MedCentral, June 6, 2022. www.medcentral.com.
37. Biles, "What More Can I Say?"
38. Ana Radovic and Megan A. Moreno, "Treatment Options for Adolescent Depression," JAMA Pediatrics Patient Page, January 28, 2019. https://jamanetwork.com.
39. Quoted in Orin Carlin, "10 Celebrities Reveal How Therapy Helped Their Mental Health," *Hello!*, May 9, 2022. www.hellomagazine.com.
40. Quoted in Andrea Michaelson, "10 Celebrities Who've Opened Up About Taking Antidepressants and Other Medications for Their Mental Health," Business Insider, July 27, 2020. www.insider.com.
41. Quoted in Kati Blocker, "ECT for Depression: Young Woman Finds Hope Through Electroconvulsive Therapy," UCHealth, February 1, 2022. www.uchealth.org.
42. Quoted in Blocker, "ECT for Depression."
43. Quoted in Children's Hospital New Orleans, "Sophia's Story: Finding Renewed Purpose in Life After Struggling with Mental Illness," News & Blog, May 2, 2023. www.chnola.org.
44. Quoted in Children's Hospital New Orleans, "Sophia's Story."
45. C. Scott Moreland and Liza Bonin, "Patient Education: Depression Treatment Options for Children and Adolescents (Beyond the Basics)," UpToDate, October 3, 2022. www.uptodate.com.

Chapter Five: Lifestyle Changes Can Help Fight Depression

46. PBS LearningMedia, "Depression: One Teen's Story," January 29, 2019. https://whyy.pbslearningmedia.org.
47. Quoted in Rachael Schultz, "Diet and Mental Health: These Women Changed Their Diets to Manage Their Anxiety and Depression," Bezzy Depression, September 1, 2023. www.bezzydepression.com.
48. Quoted in Schultz, "Diet and Mental Health."
49. Quoted in Schultz, "Diet and Mental Health."
50. Quoted in Paola Scommegna, "More Sleep Could Improve Many U.S. Teenagers' Mental Health," PRB, June 28, 2022. www.prb.org.
51. Quoted in Juliann Garey, "Teens and Sleep: The Cost of Sleep Deprivation," Child Mind Institute, November 6, 2023. https://childmind.org.
52. Marci Goldberg, "My Reason for Fighting," Anxiety & Depression Association of America, April 3, 2020. https://adaa.org.
53. Quoted in Emily Laurence, "Supplements and Non-prescription Treatments for Depression," *Forbes*, November 13, 2023. www.forbes.com.
54. Quoted in Massachusetts General Hospital, "Social Connection Is the Strongest Protective Factor for Depression," *ScienceDaily*, August 14, 2020. www.sciencedaily.com.
55. Quoted in Jon Cooper, "Stress and Depression," WebMD. July 12, 2021. www.webmd.com.
56. James Dawson, "James' Story," HeadsUpGuys, October 13, 2022. https://headsupguys.org.
57. Bliss, "Holding On."

GETTING HELP AND INFORMATION

Books

Jeffrey Bernstein, *The Anxiety, Depression & Anger Toolbox for Teens*. Eau Claire, WI: PESI, 2020.

James Chambers, ed. *Anxiety and Depression Information for Teens.* 1st ed. New York: Infobase, 2020.

Leanne Currie-McGhee, *Crisis: Teen Mental Health at Risk*. San Diego, CA: ReferencePoint, 2024

Katie Hurley, *The Depression Workbook for Teens*. Oakland, CA: Callisto Media, 2019.

Michael A. Tompkins, *The Anxiety and Depression Workbook for Teens*. Oakland, CA: Instant Help, 2022.

Online Sources

Mayo Clinic, "Teen Depression," August 12, 2022. www.mayoclinic.org.

MedlinePlus, "Teen Depression," National Library of Medicine, December 14, 2022. https://medlineplus.gov.

Mental Health America, "Depression in Teens." www.mhanational.org.

National Institute of Mental Health, "Teen Depression: More than Just Moodiness." www.nimh.nih.gov.

Nemours TeensHealth, "Depression: What You Need to Know," August 2022. https://kidshealth.org.

Websites

American Academy of Child & Adolescent Psychiatry (AACAP)
www.aacap.org
AACAP is a professional organization for psychiatrists who treat children and adolescents. It does research, advocacy, and education. The organization's website provides resources for young people with depression and other mental health disorders as well as their families.

Child Mind Institute

www.childmind.org

The Child Mind Institute is an independent nonprofit organization that provides educational information to families on mental health disorders and learning disorders in children and adolescents.

National Alliance on Mental Illness (NAMI)

www.nami.org

NAMI works to raise public awareness, educate, and provide support for those who have mental illness and their families. The organization also has a helpline that can offer resources and support to teens.

Nemours Teens Health

kidshealth.org

Run by the nonprofit Nemours Foundation, the site offers a variety of information for teens and their families to support the wellness of the whole body, including the mind.

988 Suicide & Crisis Lifeline

https://988lifeline.org

The 988 Suicide & Crisis Lifeline provides free and confidential emotional support to people in suicidal crisis or emotional distress twenty-four hours a day, seven days a week in the United States.

Substance Abuse and Mental Health Services Administration (SAMHSA)

www.samhsa.gov

SAMHSA is a federal agency that was created to make information about and services for substance abuse and mental health more accessible. It operates a helpline for information and treatment referrals.

INDEX

Note: Boldface page numbers indicate illustrations.

alcohol, 23, 52–53
American Academy of Child & Adolescent Psychiatry (AACAP), 59
American Psychiatric Association (APA), 8
American Psychological Association, 35, 37
antidepressants, 38–39
Arnett, Will, 18

Bateman, Jason, 18
Bell, Kristen, 27
Bieber, Justin, 17–18, 37
Biles, Simone, 17, 20–21, 29, 34
Bliss, Jack, 26, 54
blood tests, 12, 13
Bonin, Liza, 44
brain chemistry, 25–26
  alcohol and, 52
  antidepressants and, 39
Briggs, Alissa, 15

cannabis, 53
Centers for Disease Control and Prevention (CDC), 17, 18, 24
Child Mind Institute, 60
Children's National Hospital, 11
Clark, Casey, 12
cocaine, 53
cognitive behavioral therapy (CBT), 35, 36
Columbia University, 53
COVID-19 pandemic, 4, 28, 31–33
  as risk factor for depression, 24
Cummings, Christopher, 28

Dawson, James, 52–53
Department of Health and Human Services, US, 30
Department of Veterans Affairs, US, 29
depression
  brain chemistry and, 25–26
  definition of, 8
  genetics and, 26–28
  as medical problem, 6–7
  prevalence among adolescents, 16
  prevalence among girls *vs.* boys, 22
  stigma associated with, 37
  supporting others with, 53
  symptoms of, in teens, 9
  types of, 9–10
  See also diagnosis; protective factors; risk factors; treatment(s)
diagnosis, 13
  blood testing and, 12
  difficulties in, 14–15
disruptive mood dysregulation disorder (DMDD), 11
dopamine, 22
Doshi, Davina, 28
Dumornay, Nathalie M., 16–17

Ecstasy, 53
Eilish, Billie, 17, 18–19, **19**
electroconvulsive therapy (ECT), 41–42
estrogen, 20, 26
ethanolamine phosphate, 12

Factor, Jamie, 4–5
fluoxetine (Prozac), 38–39
Frederick, AJ, 18
Freedman, Ben, 48

61

genetics, 26–28
Germanotta, Cynthia, 21–22
Ghoshal, Malini, 34
Girls on the Brink (Nakazawa), 20
Glover, Jenna, 32–33
Goldberg, Marci, 49
Green, Jane, 46

Hairston, Danielle, 50
Harvard Medical School, 25
Hayes, Catherine, 46–47
Hayes, Sean, 18
health professionals
   capable of diagnosing depression, 13
   finding a therapist, 40
heroin, 53

interpersonal psychotherapy, 35, 37
irritability, 9
   in disruptive mood dysregulation disorder, 11
   normal teen behavior and, 15
   in premenstrual dysphoric disorder, 12

Journal of Adolescent Health, 16
Journal of the American Medical Association, 42
Juhas, Sophia, 43–44
Justin Bieber (documentary), 17

Lady Gaga, 17, 21–22, 37
LGBTQ youth, 18, 23–24
Lyons, Matthew, 28

major depression/major depressive disorder, 9
Mandal, Konoy, 42
Massachusetts General Hospital (MGH), 50–51
Mayo Clinic, 31, 34, 41
McCarney, Meg, 11
medications, 38–39
   drawbacks of, 39–41
meditation, 48

Mental Health Clinician (journal), 10
meth, 53
mood disorder
   depression as, 8
   prevalence in girls, 20
Moore, Skylar, 45
Moreland, C. Scott, 44
Moreno, Megan A., 35
Mullen, Sandra, 9, 10
Murthy, Vivek H., 16, 31
   on risk of social media, 30

Nakazawa, Donna Jackson, 20
Nassar, Larry, 20–21
National Alliance on Mental Illness (NAMI), 60
National Institute of Mental Health, 16
National Institutes of Health, 10
National Survey of Drug Use and Health, 16
Nemours Teens Health (website), 60
Neuroscience & Biobehavioral Reviews (journal), 47
neurotransmitters, 25, 39
New York University, 15
988 Suicide & Crisis Lifeline, 60
norepinephrine, 39, 52

opinion polls. *See* surveys

Perry, Katy, 38
persistent depressive disorder, 9–10
Pew Research Center, 22
polls. *See* surveys
post-traumatic stress disorder (PTSD), 29
premenstrual dysphoric disorder (PMDD), 11–12
premenstrual syndrome (PMS), 12
Prescott, David, 51
protective factors, 45
   avoiding alcohol/recreational drugs, 52–54
   diet, 46–47
   exercise, 49–50
   having social connections, 50–51

reducing stress, 51
sleep, 48–49
PsychCentral, 12
puberty, 25–26

Radovic, Ana, 35
rapid eye movement (REM) sleep, 40
risk factors, 23–24
causes *vs.*, 24
diet and, 47
gender, 22
poor sleep as, 48
social media use as, 29–31
Rolling Stone (magazine), 19

sadness
depression *vs.*, 8
prevalence among high school students, 17
seasonal affective disorder (SAD), 10–11
selective serotonin reuptake inhibitors (SSRIs), 38–39
self-esteem, 49, 51
self-injurious behavior, 4, 10
serotonin, 22, 39, 52
Sieminski, Madison Jo, 5–6, 7, 26, 28, 29
Simone vs. Herself (documentary), 21
Smartless (podcast), 18
Smoller, Jordan, 50–51
social media
as beneficial to mental health, 31
depression in girls and, 20
as risk factor for depression, 24
stress from, 29–31
stress
meditation and, 48
reducing, 51
serotonin and, 39
from social media, 29–31
from trauma, 28–29
substance abuse, 23, 52–54
Substance Abuse and Mental Health Services Administration (SAMHSA), 60

Suicide & Crisis Lifeline (988), 60
suicide/suicidal thoughts
among LGBTQ youth, 18, 24
antidepressants and, 40–41
Sultan, Hannah Wyatt, 41–42
surveys
of LGBTQ youth on prevalence of depressive symptoms, 23–24
on prevalence of depressive episodes among girls *vs.* boys, 22
showing increase in mental disorder prevalence, 16–17

talk therapy (psychotherapy), 35–36
teens
LGBTQ, 18, 23–24
normal behavior *vs.* depression in, 14–15
sleep requirements of, 49
Thames, April, 30
Thase, Michael, 47
transcranial magnetic stimulation, **43**
treatment(s)
brain stimulation therapy, 41–42
efficacy of, 35
finding a therapist, 40
finding right treatment, 44
hospital/residential, 42–44
medication, 38–41
obstacles to, 34
psychotherapy, 35–37
Trevor Project, 23–24
Turner, Sophie, 17, 19–20, **21**

websites, 59–60
Widome, Rachel, 48
Wilson, Sylia, 16–17
World Health Organization, 15

Xanax, 53

Zapata, Kimberly, 14
Zendaya, 35

PICTURE CREDITS

Cover: Antonio Guillem/Shutterstock.com

6: Monkey Business Images/Shutterstock.com
10: Stock Unit/Shutterstock.com
14: Monkey Business Images/Shutterstock.com
19: Fred Dugit/ZUMAPRESS/Newscom
21: Photofest
23: New Africa/Shutterstock.com
27: Bangkok Click Studio/Shutterstock.com
32: Ground Picture/Shutterstock.com
36: SeventyFour/Shutterstock.com
39: Rocketclips, Inc./Shutterstock.com
43: Tribune Content Agency LLC/Alamy Stock Photo
47: Pablo Rasero/Shutterstock.com
50: Jacek Chabraszewski/Shutterstock.com
52: Ground Picture/Shutterstock.com

ABOUT THE AUTHOR

Diane Marczely Gimpel teaches British literature to twelfth graders and is a former newspaper reporter who lives in southeastern Pennsylvania. She has written a dozen nonfiction books for young readers.